Conversations

in E-Learning

Diane M. Billings, EdD, RN, FAAN

Editor

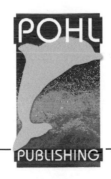

POHL

PUBLISHING

Publisher: Pohl Publishing, Inc.
312 East Nine Mile Road, Suite 11–409
Pensacola, FL 32514

Publisher: Belinda E. Puetz

Managing Editors: Patricia M. Adkison
Keleita L. (Shay) Stephens

Text & Cover Design   Susan A. Hoege
Innovative Business Communications
2910 Valley Manor Drive
Kingwood, TX 77339

ISBN 0–9717499–1–4

Printed in the United States of America.

About the Editor

Diane M. Billings, EdD, RN, FAAN

Diane is Chancellor's Professor and Associate Dean for Teaching, Learning, and Information Resources at Indiana University School of Nursing, Center for Teaching and Lifelong Learning, in Indianapolis, IN. She is an e-learner, e-educator, and e-evaluator.

Table of Contents

Section 1: *Introduction to E-Learning*

Section 2: *Strategic Planning*

Section 3: *E-Learning Tools and Platforms*

Section 4: *E-Educators*

Section 5: *E-Learners*

Section 6: *Designing Courses and Modules*

Section 7: *The Online Learning Community*

Marilyn Ryan, EdD, RN
Professor and Associate Director Graduate Programs, School of Nursing
Ball State University, Muncie, IN

Kay Hodson Carlton, EdD, RN, FAAN
Professor and Coordinator Educational Resources and Distance Learning
School of Nursing, Ball State University, Muncie, IN

Section 8: *Teaching and E-Learning*

Jane Kirkpatrick, MSN, RN
Associate Professor, School of Nursing, Purdue University, West Lafayette, IN

Cynthia Dobbs, MSN, RN, OCN
Clinical Assistant Professor, Department of Adult Health
Indiana University School of Nursing, Indianapolis, IN

Mary Lou DeNatale, EdD, MS, RN
Associate Professor, University of San Francisco, San Francisco, CA

Suzanne E. Malloy, EdD, MSN, RN
Professor, School of Nursing, San Jose State University, San Jose, CA

Sharon A. Vinten, MSN, RN,C
Clinical Assistant Professor, Department of Family Health
Indiana University, Indianapolis, IN

Roselle Partridge, MSN, RN,C
Clinical Assistant Professor, Department of Family Health, Retired
Indiana University, Indianapolis, IN

Natasha Flowers, MA
Instructional Design Specialist, Indiana University Purdue University Indianapolis
Indianapolis, IN

Section 9: *E-Quality: Evaluation, Accreditation, and Evidence for Best Practices*

Diane M. Billings, EdD, RN, FAAN
Associate Dean for Teaching, Learning, and Information Resources
Indiana University School of Nursing, Indianapolis, IN

Section 10: *Ethical/Legal Considerations*

Section I:
Introduction to E-Learning

Welcome to the world of e-learning, the use of Internet tools such as discussion forums, chat rooms, e-mail, and testing to promote learning. E-learning is the fastest growing segment of higher education and more than fifty percent of the schools of nursing in the United States are offering part or all of their courses in an e-learning format. Educators in staff development and continuing education also are using e-learning for lifelong learning. While access and convenience are the primary reasons for offering online courses, educators also use e-learning tools to facilitate teaching and learning in the classroom, and to form interactive learning communities where the best practices of the profession can be generated and disseminated. While skeptics point to concerns about high costs, changing educator and learner roles, and the lack of face-to-face interaction, the evidence indicates that learners and educators thrive in e-learning communities, and learning outcomes and expectations can exceed those of the traditional classroom. This unit will introduce the pros and cons as well as the uses of e-learning in a variety of educational settings.

Chapter 1: *What is E-Learning?*

1. *What is e-learning?*

1. E-learning is the use of Internet learning tools such as online discussion, chat, testing, and e-mail to support teaching and learning in an online community. The community may include learners, educators, and experts. The primary feature of e-learning is the opportunity for learning any time and any place in a rich and collaborative environment. E-learning is also known as Web-based learning, online learning, and Internet-based learning, and the learning environment as the online learning community or asynchronous learning network.

2. *Is e-learning the same as distance learning?*

2. E-learning is a form of distance learning because it involves separation of the educator and learner in time and space. E-learning uses the Internet as the communication delivery system in the same way that audio conferencing uses the telephone to connect learners and educators and video conferencing uses interactive video equipment and closed circuit or satellite communications systems. As the instructional technology evolves, the communication tools of traditional distance learning are merging into the e-learning environment of the Internet and will offer the best features of audio, video, and text.

3. *What do you mean by "Web presence," "Web-enhanced," and "full Web" courses?*

3. The tools of e-learning can be used to support learning in a traditional classroom or create a learning environment that is totally on the Web. *Web presence* refers to courses that have the syllabus and course information posted on a Web site. *Web-enhanced* courses are those courses that use e-learning tools to support part of the teaching and learning activities within the course; students and faculty meet face-to-face for the other class times. For example, a course on ethics in health care may meet once a week on-campus for one hour for in-class activities and tests, and then involve students in online discussions of case studies, self-testing, or sharing of drafts of papers for peer critique. *Full-Web courses*, on the other hand, never meet in a face-to-face environment. These courses use all e-learning tools to support all course learning activities. The decision to design courses as "full Web" or "Web-enhanced" depends on the purpose for offering the course on the Internet, the need for collaborative work tools, the course content, and the characteristics of the learner.

4. *I have heard the terms asynchronous and synchronous learning used in reference to e-learning; what do they mean?*

4. These terms describe how learners and other members of the learning community are interacting with each other in time. *Asynchronous* means that the interaction takes place at different times—no one is together at the same time. Asynchronous learning uses primarily discussion boards and e-mail, and allows class members to participate at a time that is convenient for them. With asynchronous learning, students and educators contribute to a discussion or take an exam at different times, but given a deadline, all work can be completed by a specified time line. Another example of asynchronous learning is self-paced learning in which learners complete assignments or modules, submit work for feedback, or take a post-test to indicate achievement of specified competencies. This type of asynchronous learning is used effectively for staff development and continuing education as it permits greater flexibility for learners who are employed and working on a varied time schedule.

Synchronous learning means that learners and educators are present and online at the same time. In an e-learning course, this occurs using a chat tool or as an Internet Relay Chat (IRC). Here, learning activities are designed to take advantage of having the input of all class members at the same time.

5. *What is the difference between an "educator-facilitated" Web course and a "self-paced" Web course?*

5. In an *educator-facilitated* course, there is an educator who is an active facilitator of the course. The educator serves as guide and coach by interacting with the course participants, is available to answer questions, guide discussion, and provide feedback, and evaluate and assess learning. Educator-facilitated courses generally have a specific start and end date.

In a *self-paced* Web course, the educator and other participants are not available on a continuous basis, although the educator may be available during specified times during the course. Here, the learner interacts with the content, uses links to resources, and obtains feedback at check points that are designed within the course. Evaluation of learning outcomes generally occurs through the use of end-of-course examinations. Self-paced courses provide learners the opportunity to study on their own time schedule.

6. What are the advantages of e-learning?

6. E-learning has many advantages for adult learners who are managing multiple responsibilities. E-learning courses and programs make learning accessible to learners who might not otherwise have access to education, particularly continuing education and post-RN degrees. E-learning courses are also convenient, because, for the most part, learners can participate at times that are convenient for them. Another advantage is that the tools that support e-learning promote active learning, collaboration, high level interaction, and rich and rapid feedback. E-learning is student-centered, promotes timely and synergistic exchange of information, and can integrate a variety of experts and best practices into the course.

7. What are the disadvantages of e-learning?

7. There are also disadvantages associated with e-learning, and learners and educators must consider these disadvantages when making decisions about teaching and learning. One disadvantage has to do with the technology, including access to it, the reliability of the infrastructure, and the learning curve required for both educators and students to become effective members of the e-learning community. Another disadvantage is difficulty using e-learning formats to teach content that is better taught in a face-to-face environment, such as teaching nursing skills or clinical practice courses.

8. What kinds of nursing courses work best for e-learning?

8. Most nursing courses can, in fact, use the strategies of e-learning. Courses that are largely "didactic" in nature, such as foundational or core courses work well in e-learning as the learning strategies involve active learning, critical thinking, and application to practice, all of which are well supported in the e-learning "classroom." Clinical practice courses can use e-learning strategies to support online "pre and post conferences," and provide access to resources for preparation for patient care. However, the actual clinical practice requires the presence of a faculty member or preceptor who is responsible for the learner and patient safety.

9. What kinds of learners are best suited for e-learning?

9. While most learners can develop "style flex" and learn in an e-learning environment, those learners who are self-directed, motivated, and are able to express themselves in reflective writing tend to be successful and have positive attitudes toward Web courses. Students who are text-based learners, as opposed to auditory learners, also tend to prefer Web courses. One positive

aspect of learning in an online learning course is the fact that learners who are normally "shy" or sit in the back of the room and are self-reflective, but do not share their thoughts with the teacher or their classmates, tend to blossom in e-learning courses.

10. Who is the audience for e-learning? Who is enrolling in e-learning courses?

10. E-learners are students, registered nurses, and healthcare professionals who are interested in advancing their education or acquiring updated knowledge, values, and skills. Academic courses and degrees (particularly RN-BSN, RN-MSN, and MSN degrees) are available on the Web. Continuing education is also offered on the Web, and there are many courses and certificate programs available in a variety of nursing specialties. E-learning is also used in staff development, primarily for the yearly "mandatories" for employment, and to teach new procedures and provide access to up-to-date and "just-in-time" learning.

11. Who are the providers of e-learning for nursing and health care?

11. There are many new providers of e-learning for healthcare professionals. These can include stand alone, degree granting schools, degree granting consortia, and non-degree granting groups such as corporate universities or publishing companies. Most schools of nursing have several or all of their courses or academic programs online. Many nursing organizations have also developed Web sites and online courses and certificate programs for their members. Drug companies, equipment manufacturers, and other commercial vendors also offer online courses to provide information about specific products. Textbook publishers and publishers of audio-visual resources use their Web sites to deliver online learning opportunities. Healthcare agencies are also providers of their own e-learning, often in a corporate environment such as corporate universities or on the internal corporate Intranet.

12. Can people really learn using e-learning strategies?

12. The answer to this question is a resounding yes! There have been many studies conducted to determine the answer to this question, and invariably the findings indicate there are no significant differences in learning outcomes between traditional classroom courses and online, or e-learning courses. The more appropriate point is that the communication tools, when used effectively by both the educator and the learner, actually facilitate learning. The evidence from research in nursing education is now showing that the opportunities for active learning, feedback, and interaction with the faculty and other participants in the course that are enabled by e-learning tools and strategies contribute to improved learning outcomes.

RESOURCES

Boettcher, J. (1999). Embracing Web learning: Faculty guide for moving courses to the Web. **http://www.cren.net**

Connor, H. (2001). Electronic education: What we know and what we do not know. *Journal of Professional Nursing, 17*(6), 273–274.

Harasim, L., Hiltz, S. R., Teles, L., & Turoff, M. (1997). *Learning with networks: A field guide to teaching and learning on-line.* Cambridge, MA: MIT Press.

Palloff, P. M., & Praft, K. (1999). *Building learning communities in cyberspace: Effective strategies for the on-line classroom.* San Francisco: Jossey-Bass.

Illinois On-line Network. **http://illinois.on-line.uillinois.edu/resources**

Chapter 2: *Staff Development Online*

1. *Why provide staff development training online versus in a traditional classroom?*

1. The "Information Age" is forcing organizations to reevaluate how training is delivered to employees. To remain viable and competitive, organizations need employees who have computer skills and possess current knowledge and skills for their job in an era when information and technology changes rapidly. How can an organization best deliver education and training to all employees? With the economic constraints facing most healthcare organizations today and in the future, online training is a viable solution to this dilemma.

Classroom training is becoming more difficult to achieve with the limited resources that staff development departments have at their disposal. Budgetary constraints of healthcare organizations typically restrict FTEs for non-direct care providers and limit ancillary department budgets that can negatively influence the amount of traditional classroom training that can be provided in an organization. The reality is that today's staff development educators in the healthcare setting do not have the luxury of standing in a classroom for hours, nor do staff have the luxury of attending classes. Staffing shortages; the need to maximize staff productivity; staff scheduling and shift work; rapid changes in health care and technology; expanding "mandatory" education requirements as directed by the Joint Commission on Accreditation of Healthcare Organizations (JCAHO), state regulations, and organizational initiatives; and merging healthcare organizations into multi-site systems are all issues that restrict the ability of staff development educators to provide traditional classroom training.

Educators must seek new methods of delivery to maximize access and flexibility of course offerings for staff, provide cost effective training, create databases/reports that track staff completion of required education programs, and efficiently assess staff competency. E-learning provides solutions to many issues facing staff development educators in the healthcare setting.

2. *What are the advantages to offering staff development training classes online?*

2. The biggest advantages are the flexibility, convenience, and access that can be realized by the staff member seeking educational opportunities. Staff can access online educational programs anytime, anywhere and the staff development department can track completion electronically, which eliminates the staff needed to manually track program completion. Advantages include:

- Quick and easy accessibility from any location

- Reduced travel time for participants

- Flexibility and convenience as to when programs are offered

- Individual self-paced learning

- Access to existing resources such as procedure or policy manuals, experts, videotapes, library services, databases, and other resource Web sites

- Reduction in program costs such as materials, handouts, manuals, room fees, food, and audiovisual equipment

- Revisions and updates to education programs are quicker and easier to accomplish online

- Easier and cheaper distribution of course materials

- Potential interactivity and communication between participants and facilitators in online courses

- Just-in-time training

- Increased quantity of courses offered online for participants to choose from to meet individual educational needs

- Immediate feedback to participants when using online testing

- Electronic tracking of participant completion and course access

- Long term cost benefits through decreased training time needed for online courses

- Increased compliance with completion of educational programs because of enhanced access and improved tracking of program completion

3. *What are the disadvantages to online delivery of staff development courses?*

3. The major disadvantages are the need for significant technological infrastructure and various Web-based training experts to support the e-learning platform and delivery. Organizations find it difficult to provide adequate computer/network access, ongoing technical support, and the experts necessary to support and create online courses. Disadvantages of online training include:

- Requires a team of experts to develop online classes,

such as instructional designer, subject matter expert, graphic designer, and information systems expert

- Increased development time needed for instructors to transform classes to a Web-based learning format

- Changes are needed to instructional delivery and methodologies to adapt to the online format

- Increased technology infrastructure and participant access to computers

- The need for learner computer knowledge/skills and an acceptance of the online method of instructional delivery

- Changes in learner participation and adaptation to new learning methods

- Technological barriers related to bandwidth and downloading times

- Security for testing online

- Lack of face-to-face interaction with the instructor and other class participants. The instructor will need to facilitate the course and monitor participant progress

- Increased costs for initial program development

- Not all courses can be delivered online

4. What would be appropriate content or types of classes to try in an online format?

4. There are very few classes that would not be appropriate for an online format for course delivery. Just as when planning a traditional class, you need to look at the instructional objectives and performance expectations students must achieve upon the completion of the training session. The instructional/performance objectives will determine the content, instructional methodologies (or interaction), and evaluation methods you use in developing the online class.

Objectives, content, and evaluation from the cognitive domain can easily be formatted online. Difficulty arises with objectives from the affective and psychomotor domain. For example, if you are teaching communication skills and participants need to role-play and visualize nonverbal communication techniques, this may be hard to accomplish online. It may also be difficult to teach a psychomotor skill online. You can put a video clip online so the student can visualize the skill, but you will not be able to evaluate a participant's competency in starting an IV if you cannot see the participant physically demonstrate the skill. However, new technology can allow visualization of skills and other participants synchronously through use of Web cameras. Use of synchronous chat rooms and asynchronous discussion boards are alternative instructional methods that can be used for online classes to engage participants in online discussion.

5. Where does an organization begin when considering implementing online training?

5. There are a number of activities that an organization should explore as part of the analysis phase in the online training development process.

- Research and define what constitutes effective, quality online training.

- Network with other organizations that have implemented online training. Learn from their successes and failures.

- Assess learners and evaluate the courses you offer. Will learners be amenable to online classes? Do you have enough users to offset the costs for online training development? Do the employees have computer skills and access to equipment? Will online training adequately assess and improve employee competency?

- Compare the cost benefit and efficacy of online versus classroom training methods. Will online training be easier, quicker, safer, less expensive, more interactive, more satisfying, and provide better learning outcomes for the participant than the traditional classroom?

- Determine the technology and expert support that will be needed by the organization to fully implement online training.

- Compare vendors for courseware/software to develop classes, learning management systems, and vendor developed online classes. Will it be cheaper to develop the classes online or purchase customizable classes from a vendor or school of nursing?

- Identify administrative and economic support required to implement online training in the organization.

6. What does an organization need to support online training?

6. Certainly the organization needs to have people resources and the appropriate team available to implement and manage Web-based training. The ideal team would include a(n):

- Webmaster to develop and maintain the education Web site on the organization's Intranet

- Project manager/educator to coordinate the team

- Instructional designer to assist with the design of the computer-based methodology of instruction

- Programmer to assist with the course authoring software/tool

- Graphic designer to create the visual appeal of the course online

- Subject matter experts to develop accurate course content

- Facilitator/educator to guide the online course, provide participant feedback, and evaluate the course/ student outcomes

- Computer systems technician to assist with service issues or technical problems

Equipment, technology, and software are other resources needed by the organization to create and distribute online classes and may include:

- An internal company Intranet to post the courses securely on the education Web site for employee only access. If the organization does not have an internal company network, a network connection to the public Internet and a Web server will be needed.

- Adequate computers that are powerful (Pentium preferred, 16 MB RAM or better) and fast enough to handle the online programs. Classes with audio and video will need fast computers to minimize the amount of time it takes to download the class. A video accelerator adapter card, a 16-bit sound card, and plug-ins are needed to run audio or video programs. If the class has animation, video or audio, the connection recommended for the end user is an ISDN or a 56 Kbps modem.

- A Web browser

- An authoring system or courseware for creating the class online. An authoring program/tool will help put the program into HTML language for use on the Web

- A learning management system or courseware that can manage aspects of the class and track student roster, student participation, successful completion, "grades," and student records.

- Adobe Acrobat is helpful when you want the organization's documents and graphics or text to be displayed in the same format no matter what computer the end user is using.

7. What are some barriers to implementing online training for staff development?

7. Because there are initial start up costs to purchase hardware and software as well as the need for information systems support, you must have administrative and economic support to implement this project. A solid business proposal must be developed that sells the concept to those who control the approval process and finances for implementing online training in the organization. The proposal should include a cost/benefit analysis between online and traditional classes, the estimated return on investment, the time savings for employees that online courses have over traditional classes, the impact on employee competency, and the efficacy of the online mode of instructional delivery on learning.

Additional barriers to implementing online courses include:

- Inadequate educator competency and computer skills to deliver courses online

- Lack of employee access to computers

- Insufficient student skill and knowledge with computer technology

- Student discomfort with the paucity of face-to-face interaction

8. How are staff learning needs assessed for online program development?

8. In the same manner as completing a needs assessment for a traditional class, a needs assessment for an online class is accomplished by:

- Identifying a training need. Data to support training needs can be obtained through interviews, focus groups, questionnaires/surveys, manager or employee requests, regulatory standards, new technology, performance improvement data, competency/work performance issues, and observation. Determine if the gap in knowledge, attitude, skill or competency/performance can be addressed through education and training or are there other factors affecting performance.

- Defining the training goal(s). Based on the identified training need(s), what do you want the learner to be able to do after participating in online training?

- Determining the existing knowledge, level, and background of the learners. Do the learners have computer skills to be able to participate in an online course? What is their current level of skill and knowledge related to the educational topic so you can create appropriate content?

9. *Is online training appropriate for all learners in the organization or are there certain learners who prefer this method of training?*

9. Not all learners in the organization will have access to computers or possess the computer skills necessary to participate in an online program. Some employees may have language barriers or learning disabilities that would make online training difficult for them. The organization must decide whether all employees will be required to participate online, or if you will need to have alternative methods of delivering educational programs to select audiences. Creating multiple methods of delivery can cut into cost and time savings of the online method. If all employees are expected to participate in e-learning, the organization will need to provide computer classes and access to computers for all employees.

Another concern is that very little research has been done on learning preferences and learning styles and their impact on success in online training. Certain types of learners may not do well with a self-directed method of learning such as e-learning. Some learners may find the isolation of e-learning difficult to adjust to without the face-to-face contact with the instructor and colleagues.

10. *Are there issues of security or confidentiality that must be addressed for online training in staff development?*

10. If you place courses on the Internet, others outside the organization will have access to these programs. Most organizations choose to place training programs on the internal company Intranet that is password accessible by employees only and typically protected behind a firewall. Healthcare organizations need to take particular care in ensuring confidentiality and security of information on their computer networks as mandated by regulatory requirements. Security policies must be in place to prevent hacker assaults, deter viruses, and prevent access to private personal information.

Intellectual property rights are a gray area when courses and information are posted on the Internet. The time, staff, and cost to create an online course needs to be considered when you post something for "free" access on the Internet. Other organizations can benefit without compensating the creators of the program. Competitors can use training information posted on the Internet to gain insight into marketing strategies and new services/technology offered. This does not make good business sense unless the organization's philosophy is to be collaborative with other healthcare entities.

Assuring testing security is another issue to address. How can you really be certain the employee who takes an online test is really the employee and doesn't "cheat" during testing? Policies should be developed that address testing security.

11. *What competencies will educators need to create training classes online?*

11. Figure 1 illustrates educator competencies for developing online courses.

Figure 1. *Educator Competencies for Developing Online Courses*

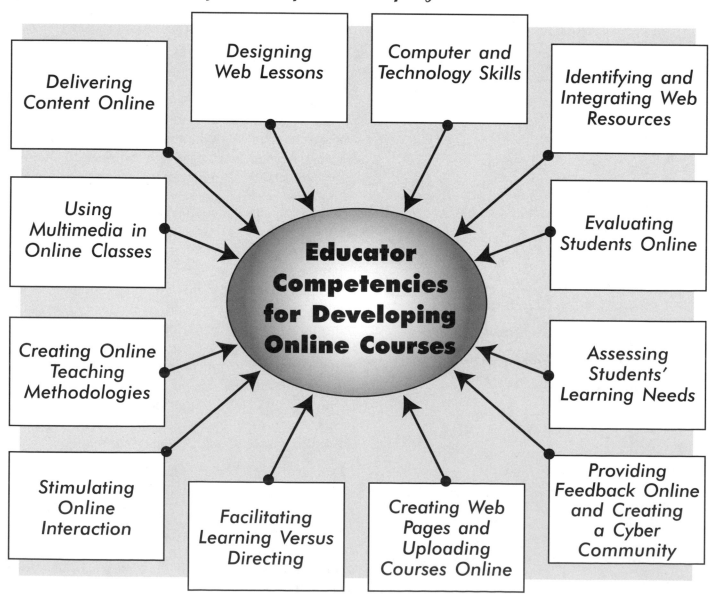

12. Can evaluation of staff competency occur online?

12. You can test learners online by administering a variety of cognitive pre or posttests (e.g., true/false, multiple choice, fill in the blank, matching, essays), observing a return skill demonstration via Web camera, assessing online discussions, or using simulations and case scenarios. One of the advantages to online testing is the immediate feedback that employees can receive. However, the true test of competency is when the employee meets the learning outcomes and actually applies the knowledge, skill, attitude, and behavior to the real work world. Verifying that a behavior change has occurred is difficult if you do not observe the actual behavior of the individual. It may help to use preceptors in the work setting to observe and validate the competency of the employee using objective performance criteria. Today technology is available to "observe" employee behavior via Web camera in the work setting by an off-site evaluator. This type of technology has been used at the University of Buffalo School of Nursing to evaluate Nurse Practitioner students at distant clinical sites.

Other methods to evaluate staff competency in the work world are employee performance review results; performance improvement or quality assurance data; quality indicators; and near miss or occurrence report information. Ideally, compare performance indicators pre and post-education intervention to determine if learning outcomes have been met.

13. What resources are available to educators for online training in the staff development domain?

13.
- Get on the Internet and look for resources! You can find everything from sample online classes, to vendors and online training consultants, how to design Web pages, professional organizations that support online training, articles on online training, Listservs, and so on.

- Read the books listed in the Resources at the end of this chapter. They are excellent resources for online training development.

- Investigate continuing education offerings or college courses on designing Web-based courses.

- Network with colleagues!

14. Can the "mandatories" be offered online?

14. Currently this is the largest use of online training in healthcare organizations and the major motivating factor behind most organizations' transition to online training.

There are several reasons why the "mandatories" lend themselves to online delivery:

- All employees must access and review the "mandatories" per the Joint Commission on Accreditation of Healthcare Organizations, Occupational Safety and Health Administration, federal, state, and individual organization standards.

- Mandatory topics required may vary depending on the job responsibilities of the employee.

- Mandatory education must occur upon hire and routinely thereafter as defined by standards or the organization.

- Specific organizational information (i.e., policies) and resources can be linked and accessed in order to customize and supplement the generic mandatory information for the organization.

- Most of the mandatory information is consistent from year to year but can be easily updated if online.

- Completion of the mandatories and online testing can be tracked electronically for the organization. This represents significant time savings for the staff development department and the manager to ensure employee completion of the mandatories.

15. How can I use online learning to simplify staff development?

15. The possibilities of online training for the organization are endless and many applications can simplify how we provide staff development. What about . . .

- Offering new employee orientation online. This eliminates the need to start employees on certain days when new employee orientation is offered or having to offer orientation multiple times in a month to accommodate staffing needs.

- Providing the mandatory education requirements online. This minimizes the need to provide multiple classes or copy and distribute volumes of written material to ensure all employees have access to the information.

- Creating a "Virtual Hospital University." Staff can pick and choose educational programs that apply to them and their job responsibilities. This means the staff development department is not tied down to set schedules for programming and employees can access programs at their convenience. Employees can have access to programs for career and professional growth opportunities.

- Testing online to eliminate the manual process of correcting tests and tracking grades.

- Tracking employee compliance with completing programs online and generating computerized compliance reports.

- Linking to internal and external resources for additional information on the program topic for the learner.

16. Should I purchase "off the shelf" staff development programs, or develop my own?

16. There are pros and cons to both purchasing vendor-created educational programming and to creating your own staff development programs. The major advantage to purchasing vendor created programs is it saves course development time, which can be very time consuming. Also educators who do not have the technical skill to develop online classes, do not have course authoring tools available to them, or the support from an instructional development team are probably better off purchasing programs. One disadvantage to purchasing vendor created programs is if content cannot be customized, the program may not be applicable to the organization. There is also a significant cost for vendor created programs on top of the annual fees the vendor charges per employee. Ongoing vendor support and viability are essential to continue to support programs that are purchased through the vendor. Another issue that you should clarify with the vendor is what platform will be needed to run the program and whether the platform is nonproprietary.

Developing your own staff development programs can ensure they are relevant to the organization's policies and standards. Although creating your own programs can save money, you will need the technical skill to create online courses, significant support from the instructional development team, and administrative support for the amount of time that must be allocated for program development.

17. If I am going to purchase staff development programs, where do I start?

17. Search for vendor advertisements in professional journals, mailings to the organization, and displays at professional conferences. Network with staff development colleagues to obtain feedback on their experiences with various vendors. Investigate the vendors that are available by reviewing their Web sites (many have sample demonstration classes online) and examine their business literature. Critique their business viability and expertise in program development.

- Have they been in business for a period of time?

- What is their client base?

- What is the economic stability of the company?

- Do they support healthcare content and who are their content experts?

- What programs do they have available and do they meet the educational needs of the organization?

- Do they outsource program development or is it created "in-house"?

- Can their programs be customized for the organization?

18. *How can I determine if the vendor of online staff development will meet my needs?*

18. Clearly articulate your needs in writing when looking at vendor support and ask the vendor for evidence that it can deliver what it says it will. Inspect the vendor's past record and call or ideally visit some of the vendor's clients. Some online training vendors have not done business with healthcare organizations, which may be a detriment if you would like to purchase vendor-developed programs. Beware some online learning management systems may not be able to be customized or support other vendors' education programs. This would require you to only purchase education programs from the one vendor.

RESOURCES

Draves, W. (2000). *Teaching on-line*. River Falls, WI: LERN Books.

Driscoll, M. (1998). *Web-based training: Using technology to design adult learning experiences.* San Francisco: Jossey-Bass.

Hall, B. (1997). *Web-based training cookbook: Everything you need to know for on-line training.* New York: John Wiley & Sons, Inc.

Webb, W. (1996). *A trainer's guide to the World Wide Web and intranets: Using on-line technology to create powerful, cost-effective learning in your organization.* Minneapolis, MN: Lakewood Books.

Chapter 3: Academic Courses and E-Learning

1. *How many nursing programs in the United States offer courses and/ or degrees for academic credit in an online format?*

1. New courses and degree programs emerge every day. It is not possible to publish here a list of these that would be current even at the moment of printing. But there are Web sites emerging that provide resources to get the prospective student started. A few of these sites are listed under "Resources."

2. *What problems might I encounter in getting academic credit for online courses taken at one university transferred to my on-campus degree program at a different university?*

2. Most universities and programs allow for the transfer of a specified number of credits from courses successfully completed at another university. Universities typically do not indicate the modality of course delivery on transcripts. Thus, the issue of course delivery should not be relevant to the decision. Course credit earned in online courses from accredited universities and programs should be transferable if within the maximum allowable transfer credit limit.

3. *Do I need special computer equipment to take an online course or degree program?*

3. Yes. All online courses use particular platforms and servers that interface with the institution's electronic infrastructure. Some universities use proprietary connection software and some simply require access to the Web. The university program typically publishes requirements for computer configurations, software, and Internet access when online courses are part of the portfolio. If this information is not readily visible in registration materials, contact the program director to get specific information. Some universities will lease compatible computers or sell them from bookstores at discount prices to students.

4. *Can I get financial aid for courses or degrees taken online?*

4. Yes. However, federal law does place stipulations on which programs qualify for financial aid. Currently there are restrictions on the proportion of the university curriculum that can be offered online or as "correspondence" courses for the university students to qualify.

5. *Do financial aid packages cover the purchase of computer equipment needed for course work?*

5. Yes. Financial aid packages can include an amount that can be used to purchase computer equipment. It is important that the program demonstrate that the purchase

of a personal computer is required of students for this to qualify for financial aid.

6. *I have heard that online courses require more student time to complete requirements than do traditional classroom-based courses. Is this true?*

6. There are misconceptions by some students that online courses are either easier or more difficult than traditional classroom formats. Typically, students without prior experience with online course work enter with a belief the course will be "easier" than a classroom format. This is perhaps due to the "ease" of access and the opportunity to do the work "anytime, anywhere" that the student has a computer and time. This flexibility does not replace the rigor of the course requirements.

When a student takes a well-designed online course for the first time, he/she is often struck by the rigor of the requirements and the time needed to complete assignments. While this should not be more time than required in any other format, the discrepancy between preconceived notions and the reality often lead to the misconception about time commitment.

7. *Do online courses really provide the same quality as classroom-based courses?*

7. Some research has demonstrated that online learning formats produce better synthesis of material and student products than the traditional classroom discussion. This is perhaps because a major feature of online courses and programs is the focus on "active learning." In the typical classroom lecture, students are passive recipients of the carefully crafted information structure of the professor. The professor does the thinking, the preparing, and the presenting of material. Students listen, take notes, and sometimes answer questions.

In the well-constructed online classroom, faculty will provide very extensive learning architectures that require students to engage fully in the material. The architecture may include a variety of modalities such as video streaming with voice and image of the professor, references for students to review, guided questions, collaborative group projects, case scenarios, and asynchronous threaded discussions. In threaded discussions, all students participate and get feedback from faculty and peers. This feature alone provides all students with the incentive to be well prepared for discussion every time, to extend their intellectual reach among their peers, and to develop projects they are proud to share with everyone in their virtual discussion group.

8. *Do these "active learning" methods lead to better quality?*

8. There is no question that we need more educational research in this area, especially related to how learning methods may or may not facilitate particular learning styles. However, many student satisfaction surveys indicate that students learn as well in traditional and Web-based formats.

9. Will getting a degree from an online program hurt my chances for admission to on-campus programs for advanced degrees?

9. The most important factors in the acceptance of courses, programs, and degrees by employers and other universities are the quality and reputation of the institution and its graduates. Quality and reputation stem from a number of factors including regional and professional accreditation, quality of the faculty and curriculum, and accomplishments of graduates. Prospective students should consider these factors in choosing online courses and programs just as they would any program. Before choosing an online program, prospective students should engage in as thorough a review of the institution as they would when applying to any degree-granting institution.

10. Why should I consider an online course or program if I have access to an on-campus classroom program?

10. While online courses and programs do provide better access to many, this is not the only or even the most important reason to consider this option. Because of the "active learning" approach of the online programs, many students find the course work more challenging and gratifying than in the traditional classroom. Also, because all students participate in most online discussion groups, feedback by faculty is usually tailored and consistent.

Some other factors to consider in making a choice for online courses are your readiness to engage in independent learning, willingness for feedback and engagement with others in the virtual space, and your ability to adapt to new methods and technologies. Part of the adaptability includes handling the inevitable frustrations of technologies in evolution. Even the most sophisticated delivery systems for Web-based formats have drawbacks and "down times."

11. How do I know which online degree programs are high quality?

11. It is critical to remember that all learning formats are subject to the same scrutiny and rigorous evaluation by accrediting agencies and other overseers. Online programs should make available to applicants their credentials of approval including institutional and state board approvals, accreditations, and information about faculty qualifications and graduate profiles.

12. Don't online courses interfere with socialization among student peers and faculty?

12. Teachers who are experienced with online virtual discussion groups find that the quality of social interaction is different than in the traditional classroom. In the virtual discussion group, all students are typically required to participate. This gives all students the opportunity to increase their facility at group discussion and allows students to get to know one another through their exchange of ideas. But disclosure is often different in virtual reality than in the face-to-face arena. It has been noted that student responses in online discussions often have greater depth and reflection than in-class responses.

Many nursing programs that offer a substantial proportion of courses online require that the students get together in "real life" for planned events and discussions. These face-to-face meetings often occur in an "intensive" format over a few days or weeks at specific intervals during the program. More educational studies need to be done to gain better understanding of how these processes differ and affect the overall social development of professionals. This is particularly important for professions in which human interaction is a significant attribute.

13. Many on-campus programs are using computer-assisted learning in course work. How much online, Web-based activities are required for a course to be listed as offered "online" in university registration material?

13. There is a great deal of variability among universities and programs about what constitutes an "online" course and how these are identified and listed in registration materials. Some of this relates to how the university is organized for delivering Web-based education. As with any course or program, prospective registrants should contact the faculty member or program director regarding questions about format and course/program requirements.

14. I have heard that online degree programs cost more than on-campus programs. Is this true?

14. Tuition among programs is quite variable. In part, this relates to the basic tuition structure of the parent university. For example, private universities and colleges tend to charge substantially more tuition than state-supported institutions. However, data indicate that the greatest growth in online development has occurred in the public sector.

The costs associated with courses and programs that heavily rely on electronic infrastructure depend on many factors. Many of these factors are outside the control of the academic institution. For example, the type of infrastructure for transmission of video content available to the university within the geographic region is one significant factor. Regional cost structure for telephonic communication is another variable factor. When constructing a tuition model, these external costs are as important as the internal factors within the university.

Within a university, there is a steep investment curve during the development phases of an online program. The financial investment relates to hardware and software purchases necessary to adapt to the program growth as well as to adapt to the specifications of the regional communication networks. In addition, faculty development and multimedia support staff must be part of the investment to ensure quality programming. Once a program is up and running, there are recurring costs associated with technical upgrades and ongoing program improvements including faculty development. It is important for students to weigh the trade-offs of increased tuition costs with access, convenience, and overall quality of the program.

15. *How do I know that academic materials, including papers, tests, and grades, delivered via the Web are confidential?*

15. Confidentiality is of considerable concern with all Web-based activity including in education, commerce, or health care. Institutions that conduct business on the Web develop internal confidentiality methods. One method, referred to as a "firewall," is network software that "authenticates" the users as valid. The "firewall" may include dedicated, unique servers for course and program use not accessible to unauthorized program personnel. It may also include the use of passwords as well as message encryption for added security.

Today, there are no "fire proof" methods to ensure absolute confidentiality for material transmitted via the Web for any use. However, this is also true for most information stored in paper format and transmitted via regular or intra-institutional mail or facsimile. Prospective students may want to question program officers about the methods employed by that institution to ensure or promote confidentiality.

16. *If I develop a paper for academic credit and submit it to my faculty via the Web, is it copyright protected?*

16. Copyright protection laws in the United States apply to all material in this country regardless of vehicle of publishing or transmission. Copyright protection exists with the caveat that the author can verify or prove ownership of the ideas or publication. Thus, students should always retain a copy of papers submitted, regardless of transmission vehicle, to verify ownership of the material.

RESOURCES

Potempa, K., Stanley, J., Davis, B., Miller, K. L., Hassett, M. R., & Pepicello, S. (2001). Survey of distance technology use in AACN member schools. *Journal of Professional Nursing, 17*(1), 7–13.

http://chronicle.com/infotech

http://www.wordwidelearn.com/medical-education.htm

http://www.nu.edu/featured/nursing.html

http://on-linegraduateschool.tripod.com/health.htm

http://www.allnursingschools.com/find/

Acknowledgment: The author thanks Katherine O'Meara, PhD, RN, for her thoughtful review of and feedback on this manuscript.

Chapter 4: *Continuing Education Online*

1. What is continuing education (CE) online?

1. CE online is just a method of accessing a continuing education offering via a Web site. You interact with the content by reading or interacting in some way, and in most cases, you must take some kind of test and/or complete some type of evaluation form before you are awarded contact hours. The advantages include instant access 24 hours a day, 7 days a week, to a wide variety of content. Most CE offerings have a test that is graded instantly, and a certificate that can be printed as soon as you successfully complete the program. The only real disadvantages are those related to a lack of comfort using and navigating the World Wide Web.

2. What different kinds of CE will I find online?

2. The most common kind of CE online offerings are articles from a journal accompanied by a test. This is really just an alternate delivery system of the same content you can read in the journal. Other types include:

- Webcasts—a presentation by a speaker that can be seen and heard on a computer screen. Often the live presentations are archived and can be viewed any time after the event is over.

- Case studies—some that provide interactivity throughout the case; others that just ask some questions after reviewing all the material.

- Short courses—which can provide up to 15 hours of CE credit. Some current topics include writing for publication and test development. Longer courses are also available, but they generally award academic credit rather than contact hours.

- Multimedia—more and more CE offerings are incorporating multimedia elements like animations and video clips into the content. Audio segments might include heart and lung sounds or an expert delivering a lecture with Power Point slides. In some cases you can interact with an image or a model to get more information. As connection speeds improve, expect to see more and more multimedia online!

3. How can I find online CE?

3. Check the Web sites of nursing organizations. Most of the larger organizations have online versions of their journals with CE offerings and also provide lists and links to other sources of CE on the Web. Publishers of nursing information often have CE on their Web sites.

Nursing portals, like **allnurses.com**, provide extensive lists and links to CE sites. Other general portals and search engines like Yahoo and Google have directories. You can work through a number of menus and submenus in the Health or Medical sections of their directories. There you may find "nursing" listed, and within the nursing category may be a list of sites providing CE. In Google, the trail would be Health>Nursing>Education> Continuing Education.

4. Can I use a search engine to find an online course?

4. Sure! This can be especially useful if you are looking for CE on a specific topic. Enter (name of topic) and the term "continuing education." Example: "pheochromocytoma" and "continuing education." You might also want to add the word nursing to the list of search terms. Check the help section for the search engine to make sure that you are entering terms correctly and that you are using the appropriate symbol for a phrase. A few search engines, like Alta Vista, let you use the NEAR command, which indicates that the terms must be within a few words of each other.

5. How can I tell if it is a good course?

5. If the name of the organization or company that is responsible for the Web site is not one that you recognize, there are other things you can check.

- First check the provider status. There should be a statement that goes something like this… (Name of Web site or company) is accredited as a (provider or approver) of continuing education in nursing by the (name of accrediting body). Many providers use the American Nurses Credentialing Center's (ANCC) Commission on Accreditation. Specialty organizations may have their own accreditation bodies.

- Read through the list of authors. Do you recognize any names?

- Sample a CE offering. Many sites let you read at least one offering for free. Use your judgment to determine if the depth is appropriate for your needs. Is there too much or too little detail?

- Ask yourself if there is any possibility of bias in the information. If a company is selling a product, you might be wary that it is not providing as much information on competing products or treatment approaches.

- Finally, check to see if there is a name and address of the company and some information about the owners. If not, cross it off your list!

6. What are some features to look for in online CE?

6. Let's face it, most of us do CE online because it's time to renew our nursing license and we're still a few credits short. So some of the most important features are those that make it easy to complete the CE activity quickly and obtain that needed certificate immediately. These features include

- Payment options: Most of you will want to pay online with a credit card (I'll talk about the safety of paying online in another question). But for those who are still wary of putting a credit card number in a Web site form, check to make sure that the Web site offers other payment options.

- Ability to print a CE certificate as soon as you complete the offering

- A customer service telephone number or other method of contacting a real human being in case you encounter some technical difficulty. Some Web sites have a customer service representative available in an online chat room!

- A reasonable failure policy. Many sites will let you take the CE test a second time for free or for a reduced fee if you fail it the first time.

- Access to content. Suppose you begin a CE offering but cannot complete it in one sitting because you lose the Internet connection, the baby is crying, you fall asleep at the keyboard, or some other emergency crops up. A good CE site will allow you to get back into that CE program just where you left off, saving you considerable time and effort.

- Record-keeping: For those who do their CE well in advance of licensure or certification renewal dates, what happens if you misplace your certificate? Good CE sites will provide an easy way for you to print out a second certificate by giving you access to the list of CE offerings you have completed. But remember, features like this require you to remember your user name and password so that you, and only you, can access your record. But have no fear if you forget your password. A good site will offer reminders to help you recall your password. If you still can't remember it, a good site will have a quick and simple process to send it to you or assign you a new password via an immediate e-mail message.

7. How are CE hours determined?

7. CE hours are determined by the amount of time the individual interacts with the content. Most CE providers and approvers like the American Nurses Credentialing Center (ANCC), the American Association of Colleges of Nursing (AACN), and the International Association for Continuing Education and Training (IACET) award one contact hour or other CE unit or credit for each 50 to 60 minutes of interaction with the content, including the time it takes to complete the test and/or evaluation form. If you attend a conference session of 75 to 90 minutes, you would receive 1.5 contact hours. If you access that same session via a Web cast, the hours would be the same. When the content is in text, the people who develop the content conduct a pilot test by sending the material out to approximately 10 people who read it and take the test, then report how long it took them to complete. The average amount of time that it takes 10 people becomes the number of contact hours awarded.

8. How much does online CE cost?

8. Online CE currently ranges from $3.00 to $40.00 a credit, but some offerings are free! Expect to pay a little more for multimedia formats and for content from well-known experts. Free CE is often developed with a grant from a pharmaceutical company or an equipment manufacturer that is eager to have nurses think kindly about its products. If it is a reliable Web site (see the answer to the question "How can I tell if it's a good course?" above), then the company paying for CE development will have no editorial control over the content, except, perhaps, to specify the topic. Take advantage of some of the freebies if the content meets your needs!

9. Is it really safe to pay online?

9. If you have already determined that a known accreditation body awards the contact hours and you are satisfied with the quality of the CE, then you are dealing with a reputable site. The site should provide some reassurance regarding safeguards for how it handles credit card transactions. Most sites just immediately connect to a transaction-processing server that verifies the card number and deposits the payment in a merchant bank account. Most of these use the same security that banks use to transfer funds from place to place. And most CE sites do not keep a record of your card number. Some browsers use a symbol (like a lock) in the lower left-hand corner of the screen that indicates a secure site. Others provide a message in text on the screen.

Look for something to ease your concerns, but think, is it any less risky to give your card number to a waiter in a restaurant or your card number to an individual over the telephone?

10. *I am the director of staff development in a large hospital. Can the hospital contract with an online company and pay for CE for nurses?*

10. Yes, several companies offer large libraries of CE content and the opportunity for an agency to purchase CE for employees. Generally there is a considerable discount on the price per CE credit and the company also provides record keeping of employee names and courses taken.

11. *What if I want to create my own online CE?*

11. A few companies provide tools for making simple online CE courses on your own. But remember, making your own CE course is not that easy. You need skill with several different types of software and LOTS of time! Read Chapters 8 and 9 in this book to learn more about learning management systems and the tools for creating and managing content. Then read Chapter 20, which covers layout and design issues before you commit to creating your own CE course. But if you have the skills and/or access to people with the skills that you need, go for it! It can be a wonderfully challenging and rewarding experience and a lot of fun too!

Section 2:
Strategic Planning

Developing and offering e-learning courses and programs is resource intensive. Before you begin your adventures in e-learning, you must have a sense of direction, sufficient resources, and a supportive organizational culture. A strategic plan is essential for identifying direction and resources, and initiating the dialogue that must occur at every level of the organization. In this unit you will learn how to develop a strategic plan, an internal marketing plan, and an e-learning marketing plan.

Chapter 5: *Strategic Planning*

1. *What is a strategic plan for e-learning?*

1. A strategic plan for e-learning is a guide to identifying the resources needed to offer online modules, courses, or programs. The plan is a mechanism by which educators identify their mission and goals for e-learning, identify the required resources, establish a timeline, and develop a business plan to support the entire project.

2. *Why develop a strategic plan?*

2. Having a strategic plan serves several purposes. First, the process of developing the plan will assist you to establish goals and outcomes, and think through how you are going to achieve the intended outcomes. However, the most important reason for making a plan is to identify the resources you will need and to be sure all of the resources are in place so that you and the institution are positioned for success. Other reasons to develop a strategic plan include providing background detail for grants or funding sources, and showing administrators and decision makers that you have thought through what is needed and that you are serious about developing an online course/program. The plan may also reveal that the organization is not ready to proceed, or that e-learning does not fit with the mission of the organization. Finally, the plan can be used as a guide to evaluating outcomes.

3. *What are the elements of a strategic plan?*

3. The strategic plan should be logical and communicate your plans to the audience. If the organization uses a strategic planning process, use that one. A strategic plan is also similar to a business plan or an economic model, and the organization may use this approach to project planning. Table 1 illustrates essential elements of a planning process.

Table 1. *Elements of the Planning Process*

Mission and vision for the project	Describe the mission and vision; relate it to the mission and vision of the organization.
Project description	Describe concisely.
Goals and timelines	Identify several goals; indicate specific timelines for accomplishing each goal.
Target audience	Identify learners; describe who they are; describe their geographic location. Indicate numbers of learners to be served by the course or module.
Course design and development plan	Describe how the course will be developed. Who will be the content authors? How long will it take to develop? Will the course be "full Web"? Teacher-facilitated? What course development and management tools will be needed? How many courses will be developed throughout the project?
Personnel	Identify all personnel required to support the project.
Technical resources	Identify all resources including those existing and those needed to be acquired.
Financial plan	Develop a plan indicating costs, both direct and indirect costs.
Marketing plan	Develop an internal and e-learning marketing plan (see Chapters 6 and 7).
SWOT analysis	Identify Strengths, Weaknesses, Opportunities, and Threats as they relate to the project.
Evaluation plan	Indicate how you will measure the outcomes of the project.
Recognition and reward structure	Develop a plan describing how educators will be encouraged, recognized, and rewarded for being innovators.
Success or exit strategy	Establish expectations for use of the course by learners, the "break even point." Describe the benefits and losses you can withstand. Consider the risk factors you will face and how you will determine when to "exit" from offering e-learning courses, if needed.

4. Exactly what resources will I need to start developing and offering an e-learning course or program?

4. Getting started, and then continuing to offer e-modules, courses, or programs is a resource-intensive effort. Be sure to identify all of the resources *before* you get started. These resources may overlap; you may already have access to these resources or may need to purchase others; and in the case of personnel on the instructional team, often one person can assume several roles. Also, keep in mind that the cost associated with these resources will decrease as you develop more courses and obtain experience and efficiency in developing and offering e-learning programs (see Section 3).

Infrastructure: servers; workstations for educators and developers; Web site; learning management system software; course development software; registration data bases; e-commerce software and capability to conduct online business and registration transactions.

Personnel: network administrators, educators, developers; instructional designers; librarians or resource specialists; content experts (educators); programmers, graphic artists, copyright specialists; marketing department; secretarial assistance.

Learner support: Technical assistance (Help Desk); orientation programs; computer laboratories (or require learners to have access to a computer); desktop access (see also Section 5, Chapter 16).

5. What is an instructional team?

5. Unlike teaching in the classroom which tends to be rather private and even solitary, e-learning uses a team approach bringing together needed resources to develop the best course possible. The role of the educator, when working with this team, is to coordinate the content expertise as well as the pedagogical, technological, and ethical/legal expertise. Online courses are best developed with the support of a team with both technical and pedagogical expertise.

6. Do all members of an instructional team need to be in place before I start developing an e-learning course or program?

6. Although it is possible to start with few resources, the course will be better developed and implemented if most of the roles of the instructional team can be filled. A common mistake is to think that an enthusiastic educator or Web specialist can develop a Web course. If you have limited resources, I suggest an instructional designer, a Web programmer, and a content expert to start with.

7. How much does it cost to develop e-learning courses/programs?

7. E-learning requires a substantial investment in resources, and the investment in resources must be offset by benefits such as fiscal return on investment, service to users, or contribution to the overall mission of the organization. When estimating costs, you must include indirect infrastructure costs as well as direct costs of course development, educator development, ongoing course facilitator/teacher, learner support, and marketing. For some organizations, developing e-learning offerings is viewed as a business venture, and they plan on two to three years of investment before generating revenue.

There are several methods for calculating costs of developing online courses and programs noted in the resource section of this chapter. Although each organization should estimate its own costs using formulae for infrastructure and personnel costs, a general estimate is that it can cost about $25,000 to develop one 3-credit academic course.

8. Where can I find funding to develop online courses?

8. Adequate funding must be secured prior to developing an e-learning course or program. Often a single course is developed from the good will and enthusiasm of a single educator as a pilot test, but adequate funding will be needed to sustain the efforts. Funding can be obtained from an operations budget, grants, or contracts.

Begin the search for funds by looking within the organization for sources of support, either contributed or budgeted. If the institution is not able to make a financial commitment to support e-learning development, then it is unlikely you will be able to convince external sources to support your efforts. Next, explore possibilities for funding from state and federal granting agencies as well as private foundations and organizations. Partnerships are also opportunities to share and leverage scant resources. Most colleges and universities have small grant programs to stimulate faculty to develop online courses; healthcare agencies may also have funds to support course development. Also explore the possibility of funding from state workforce development grants. Higher education commissions are often seeking to develop a suite of courses for their online consortia, and your content may meet their funding guidelines. Partnering with a vendor of online education is also a possibility as these vendors are often seeking additional content to offer on their platforms. Many of these and other funding sources can be located by conducting an online search.

RESOURCES

Boettcher, J. (1999). *Embracing Web learning: Faculty guide for moving courses to the Web.* **http://www.cren.net**

Morgan, B. (2000). *Is distance education worth it? Helping to determine the cost of online courses.*
    http://www.marshall.cdu/~morgan16/onlinecosts/

Technology Costing Methodology Project. **http://www.wiche.edu/telecom/projects/tcm/**

Teaching Learning Technology Group. **http://www.tltgroup.org**

Chapter 6: *Internal Marketing*

1. What do you mean by "internal marketing"?

1. Marketing is a systematic approach to analyzing, planning, implementing, and evaluating programs for the purpose of establishing beneficial exchanges between individuals and groups to achieve organizational objectives. Internal marketing refers to communicating with key constituents within the organization; it is a specific and planned process to inform those who will be affected by the decision to offer Web-based courses. Because the use of e-learning is new and requires organizational commitment, it is important to consider who within the organization needs to be informed, and how. Internal marketing is a starting point for discussions about e-learning within a department or organization.

2. Why is it important to market e-learning within my organization?

2. Developing e-learning courses and programs will involve just about everyone in the organization, and will result in extensive and long-lasting change. Since these changes will have an impact on fiscal and human resources, individuals and groups within the organization need to be a part of the planning process.

3. Who are the internal audiences I need to consider?

3. Begin first with the learners or users of e-learning courses or modules; their needs must be identified along with their readiness to be e-learners (see Section 5, Chapter 17). You will also need to consider departmental colleagues who will be involved with e-learning, because once one Web course is available, other courses will follow, and teaching colleagues should be ready for this possibility. Education directors, administrators, and financial officers must also be involved with planning for e-learning from the outset. Of course, you will be working with a technical support team or contracted technical services; these individuals are essential to success and must work with you from the beginning. Finally, do not forget the marketing department, the Web site manager, and others who are responsible for representing the organization to external constituents.

4. How do I "do" internal marketing?

4. Internal marketing is a planned process. The strategic plan (see Chapter 5) can serve as the basis for the dialogue with key players within the organization who must be involved from the start. Identify existing forums for discussion such as curriculum committees or educational planning boards as a natural starting point for internal marketing. Once consensus is obtained from the immediate work group, proceed through organi-

zational channels. Ask as you go, "Who else should I discuss this with?"

It is also helpful to think of internal marketing as planned change. Begin with goals and clear outcomes, and identify points of support as well as points of resistance along the way to implementing the strategic plan. One of the purposes of internal marketing is to develop appropriate strategies to manage the barriers and facilitators of change.

5. *What are some "tips" for preparing an effective internal marketing plan?*

5. Each organization has its own "culture" and you will want to develop the internal marketing plan accordingly. Start internal marketing before initiating any action. Communicate early and often with those who will be most affected by the start up of an e-learning course or program. Develop a strategic plan that shows benefits as well as risks, and engage each group in a discussion of these benefits and risk as they pertain to them. Another strategy is to start small and consider the first e-learning efforts as a "pilot project." It is also helpful to start with educators who are enthusiastic and already excited about e-learning, and will be positive spokespeople throughout the organization. Do not forget to identify reward structures that will entice the "innovators" to continue and others to join in. These others may include merit raise promotion and tenure committees, department chairs, and administrators.

6. *How do I handle organizational resistance?*

6. The first step is to identify why individuals or the organization itself are resistant. It is helpful to seek reasons for resistance and identify points of negotiation. Offer information that is specific to the needs of the organization and seek opportunities to explain the benefits that would accrue to the organization. Use the strategic plan to show concrete goals and anticipated outcomes. If finances are a concern, indicate potential sources of fiscal support. Finally, you may need to accept the fact that e-learning is not a match with the organization's mission or a fit with priorities for fiscal resources at this time. Without the support of the organization, it will be impossible to launch an e-learning project of any scope.

7. *How can I help the supervisor/department chair/dean understand the time and resources it takes to develop a Web course?*

7. Part of the internal marketing plan is to indicate the resources needed and where they will come from. Course development is a large initial resource outlay; it requires a substantial amount of time to develop Web courses. Course development time is estimated as much as 30 hours for each contact hour when the course involves extensive programming.

Internal marketing provides an opportunity to convince administrators just what is needed to undertake developing and offering Web courses. The strategic plan indicates the extent of this support. Administrators must understand that success will require the needed support or ways to adapt in an environment without it. Again, open communication and discussion are important.

8. How can I be a champion for e-learning in the organization?

8. The "risk takers" or "innovators" or "early adopters" within an organization who are interested in developing Web courses often end up being the "internal marketers" or "champions" for e-learning. Administrators and co-workers look to these champions for accurate information to make informed decisions. If you end up becoming this "champion," it is helpful if you gather information, evaluate your experiences, provide data, and give credible testimony about the e-learning strategic plan for the organization. Then, look for formal and informal forums to share this information. These forums may include departmental meetings, staff meetings, or curriculum committees. Methods can include reports, presentations, "water cooler conversations," and even notices in the organization's e-mail or newsletter.

As the "e-learning guru" in the organization you will be able to provide facts, inform others of your own experiences (both positive and negative), and assist others to find appropriate resources. You will become the keeper of the internal marketing plan and use your expertise to assist others, as the organizational commitment to e-learning becomes a reality.

9. How can I help the organization recognize success?

9. Internal marketing also involves recognizing accomplishments. Use existing communications channels such as "Employee of the Month," teaching awards, merit recognition, internal newsletters, and e-mail distribution lists to recognize "stars." You may also consider creating new recognition vehicles such as certificates of appreciation or new teaching awards. One dean held a luncheon to recognize the Web teachers at the school. Finally, do not forget to work with members of merit review, career ladder, or promotion and tenure committees to help them understand the scholarly nature of developing and teaching Web courses.

RESOURCES

Abruzzese, R. S. (1996). *Nursing staff development: Strategies for success* (2ⁿᵈ ed.). St. Louis: Mosby.

Draves, W. A. (1998). *Marketing online courses, seminars, and conferences*. Manhattan, KS: Learning Resources Network (LERN).

Kelly Thomas, K. J. (1998). *Clinical and nursing staff development: Current competence, future focus* (2ⁿᵈ ed.). Philadelphia: Lippincott.

Chapter 7: *Marketing E-Learning*

1. What do you mean by marketing e-learning?

1. Marketing has ceased to be the "m" word in education. We now recognize that we must help people understand what we have to offer them—and that involves using marketing strategies to reach out and persuade. Marketing savvy is especially important in e-learning for two reasons: competition among educational providers and uncertainty among students about online learning. A daunting number of e-learning competitors are out there—both public and private organizations—vying for students. Some e-educators will prevail while others will back away when they fail to make e-learning work for students and the institution. Right now, many students are still unfamiliar with e-learning or hesitant to try it. We need to inform, inspire, and encourage them to try something new.

2. What is the difference between marketing and advertising?

2. When people think of marketing, they usually think of ads and TV commercials. In fact, the promotion you see is just the tip of the iceberg of marketing activity. A great deal of research and planning needs to go on below the surface to create the match among product, market, and message. Everybody seems to have an 80–20 rule. Here's a 40–40–20 rule that marketers offer: success in marketing is based 40% on quality product, 40% on the right market, and 20% on creative promotion. The lesson is this: if you haven't done your homework first, attractive (and expensive) advertising won't make a program successful. You first need to do the research to ensure that you are meeting learners' needs with a product (e.g., course, program). Then you need to study the target market—how to reach it and how to talk to it. Based on this careful research, you build the marketing plan. After the strategy is well defined, graphic design, copy writing, and sales skills finally come into play.

3. You say research comes before marketing planning. What do we need to do?

3. Make a commitment: No "data-free" decisions. Once you and the organization commit to data-informed strategic marketing planning, you're half-way there. Here's a simple example: the people answering the phones report lots of calls from Virginia. The director says, "let's beef up our advertising in Virginia—there seems to be a market there." Before you act, you verify the "hunch" via the inquiry database. If, in fact, there has been no significant upward trend in inquiries from Virginia, you will question whether advertising dollars

would be well spent in a Virginia campaign. To move away from "data-free" decision-making, the first task is to establish ready access to your own institutional data. Get to know your customer base (i.e., current and past students and those who have inquired) both demographically and psychographically.

4. What's meant by primary and secondary research?

4. Lab experiments and surveys are examples of primary research—original data gathering. Secondary research involves identifying and using information others have gathered. This is a valuable ($$!) distinction. When you find marketing questions you need to answer, you can often save a lot of time and money by looking around for existing information. Data are all around us. The challenge is to locate it. Ask yourself who else might have needed information about, for example, the nontraditional student market in Indianapolis? Who keeps information about the age of students, their places of employment, their geographic locations? Ask yourself what can I infer from looking at my own customer data? Is there marketing information to be gleaned from instructor or course evaluations?

5. When do I need primary research as opposed to secondary research?

5. When you need specific information that no one else will have, you need primary research, BUT I strongly suggest that you exhaust the possibilities for secondary research before you commit to primary research. Even if you decide on primary research, it doesn't necessarily have to be elaborate. This research can be anything from a simple focus group or quick e-mail survey to an in-depth study.

6. Can we do our own research or do we need to contract with someone else for it?

6. A key to doing good research is knowing the right questions to ask. You may want to seek out a colleague at the institution who knows research methodology. Have a talk about what you *think* you want to know. Once you're sure primary research is called for and once you've defined the questions, you'll know better whether you can handle the research in house or not. Be sure to give yourself credit for your own grasp of the question at hand. Remember that anyone you bring in from the outside will have to be educated about the organization and the particular issue you're looking into. Even if you outsource the research, you will invest a fair amount of your own time and resources.

As with any investment, you'll need to look at the

7. What are some basic research methods we can implement ourselves?

potential payoff. If you spend $10,000 on research to get a million dollar program headed in the right direction, it will be money well spent.

7. A good marketer is always testing something. You begin to think in spreadsheet form! It's an occupational hazard. But market research is not all number crunching. There are informal and qualitative methods as well as quantitative ones. Carefully implemented pilot projects are also a form of research.

I define research broadly to include day-to-day anecdotal research—the feedback from the front-line phone staff, spontaneous student comments, the institutional wisdom offered by longtime staff, the articles you read, the tips and trends you pick up at meetings and conferences. If you're committed to data-informed marketing, you're always on the alert for relevant information. Other soft research methods include focus groups, intelligence gathering through the Internet, executive interviews, advisory groups, and SWOT (Strength, Weaknesses, Opportunities, Threat) analyses.

Let me describe some types of quantitative research. Research should always include analysis of institutional data, revealing such things as inquiry and enrollment trends, conversion rates, and customer profiling. The institution's Web site will offer stats reflecting customer preferences and problems with the functionality of the site. Simple surveys can be conducted by e-mail or on the Web site. (We're finding that busy professionals sometimes respond better to course evaluations they can submit electronically.)

Tracking the responses to course or other promotions is critical as you look at cost effectiveness of activities. But it's complicated these days, when customers can contact us in person, by phone, in snail mail or e-mail, by fax, and on the Web! Nevertheless, sleuthing out the response to promotional efforts is critical to figuring out how successful various marketing efforts have been—and for fine-tuning them for next time.

Finally, don't forget the expeditionary or pilot project. (Failure can be a research finding!) If you're about to launch something big, consider designing and assessing it first as a pilot project.

8. *What is integrated marketing?*

8. This "hot" term has been tossed about in recent years, with numerous definitions. Broadly, it refers to integrating marketing planning with the organization's strategic planning and developing a customer orientation throughout the organization. If you practice integrated marketing, planning is horizontal, not dictated from the top. That means *everybody* needs to think marketing—it can't be a peripheral activity or an afterthought. (Have you heard this? "Oh, by the way, I have a new program coming up in 6 weeks and I need a brochure!")

And *everybody* needs to think customer service. Remember, it's cheaper to retain current customers (through excellent service and quality programming) than to cultivate new ones.

Integrated marketing also refers to an integrated image. Materials and messages need to be coherent and recognizable over time. And here's an important tip: institutional affiliation is probably the thing that most distinguishes you from your competitors. Be sure that your affiliation is obvious in all print and electronic publications.

9. *How can the entire organization get involved in marketing?*

9. The person(s) responsible for marketing should participate in strategic planning. That way marketing plans are consistent with the goals of the organization, and market research can help inform strategic planning. As you craft marketing plans, create a continuous feedback loop among program directors and other stakeholders. You benefit from the creativity of lots of people and secure their buy-in for the plans.

As for customer service, you might start by developing a "customer contact" list—identifying all the points at which a customer has contact with the organization, in person or through various media. Then set up a committee to examine the list and draft a consistent, coherent approach to customer contact. As a result, you may discover you need more staff training in customer service. You may find ways to economize on mailings and maximize customer correspondence. And here's an important point: studies show that satisfied employees generate satisfied customers. So include "front-line" staff in discussions of customer service, and show your support of that staff heartily and often.

10. What works better — ads, direct mail, or online marketing?

10. It just makes sense: People who are comfortable online are the most likely to enroll in e-learning, so there's a good match between online marketing and the e-learning market. The old wisdom still applies, however—the more often people see a message, and the more places they see it, the more likely they will be to respond. So don't skip one medium in favor of another unless you're very sure of the market.

Of course the relative effectiveness of different forms of promotion varies depending on the product and market. We're noticing that more and more inquiries are coming in via the Web and e-mail. However, we have found that, while potential students may begin with a Web search, most will eventually want printed materials.

Even though direct mail is expensive (e.g., printing, list purchase, mail preparation, postage), it's a mainstay of educational marketing and usually yields the best results. This may surprise you, but its effectiveness depends more on getting the mailing into the right hands than on the look of the piece itself. That's the 40–40–20 rule again.

Among the common modes of educational advertising, paid ads actually come in last in terms of return on the dollar—generally speaking.

11. Is there a role for a sales person?

11. If the word *sales* bothers you in relation to education, let's call this function "educational outreach." Often, successful marketing is relationship dependent. We depend on counselors and advisors to carry our message to students. We depend on word-of-mouth advertising from previous customers. We depend on employers to encourage employees to seek training. A "sales person" or "outreach coordinator" can work to build strong ties with these key people—to understand their concerns and address them in mutually beneficial ways.

This brings me to the concept of "wholesale vs. retail." At the university, we have typically promoted products to individual students or their parents—a retail approach. Using a sales or outreach approach, we can begin to sell our product wholesale. An outreach coordinator can negotiate with employers to deliver programs to employees on contract or establish links with professional associations to design custom programs or promote directly to a professional group. The varieties of partnerships and affiliations are many, and obviously economies of scale are present when you sell many products at once.

12. What special tips do you have for marketing online products?

12. Let's talk specifically about e-learning here. There are some things we know from experience:

1. E-learning is not for everybody. The completion rate for online courses typically ranges anywhere from 50% to 80 or 90% if a learning cohort is established. We need to help potential students self-select e-learning, and then we need to support them during the process.

2. Lots of people are intrigued by e-learning but also intimidated. We need to make e-learning less threatening and more familiar.

3. The big market for e-learning is working adults. Top priority for them is convenience. We must make Web sites and printed materials as straightforward and clear as possible. Application and enrollment should be offered online as well as in print. Advising should be available by toll-free phone.

4. The second most important element for adult students is service. We need to be prepared within organizations to minimize the hassle and maximize the learning experience.

5. After the dot com implosion, people are more skittish about getting involved with an online company. The brick-and-mortar schools have an important advantage—long-standing, confidence-inspiring operations. Make the most of it. Be sure the institutional affiliation is strong on the Web site and in your promotional materials.

13. What can we do to ensure repeat business?

13. Learner retention is part of an educational mission. It's also good business. The student who has a good experience with us continues to enroll and speaks favorably about us to others. Those retained students are gold. Clearly, to retain a student, a fine educational experience that meets the student's needs is paramount. Student evaluations and exit interviews help us refine our efforts along those lines. Excellent student services are also key to keeping our "gold" students. Marketers, by employing the principles of customer relationship management, can do their part to ensure student retention and generate repeat business.

14. What is customer relationship management (CRM)?

14. We all want to see students succeed. If we use technology thoughtfully, and if we create a culture of customer focus within an organization, we can tailor products and messages to customers, serve them better, and win their loyalty.

To that end, keep the student's interests and other relevant personal information in a database, and then use it to serve this student. Advise the student when a new class opens in an area of interest. Let the student elect to be part of an online newsletter distribution—or choose *not* to receive the e-mail. Remind the student when an important deadline is approaching. The possibilities go on and on.

There is a lot of exciting literature on CRM right now. Elegant software is available for managing with CRM. Whether we use CRM software or not, the principles are worth applying.

15. What technology do we need for CRM?

15. This might be the toughest question to try to address to in a few sentences! In fact, at a recent meeting of deans and educational program directors, information technology ranked as their number one challenge.

A DBA (database administrator) on staff could manage data, keeping it up to date, fully stocked, and easy to use. Most of us don't have the luxury of such a person. To become more sophisticated in the collection and use of data to serve the customer, start by taking inventory of all the places data reside in the organization. Most likely, there will be several different data stores in several different formats. When you know where they all are and what information they contain, you can decide how to make the best use of them for marketing.

Next step: determine what data you still need and how to collect them. You may decide to design a data system yourself, figuring out how to collect, enter, and use the data. Before you plunge into this, do some secondary research. Others in the facility have no doubt dealt with this challenge. Find these people and get their advice. Maybe there's even a database in use that you could adapt for your purposes! A word of caution: Beware of having a cheap custom database developed by someone who creates it and then leaves you with a beast no one knows how to house and feed.

For software to manage marketing database(s), I recommend Microsoft Access as a flexible, user-friendly program.

16. *How do we make the best use of the Web for marketing?*

16. First off, you need a top-notch site—one that's attractive, efficient, and accessible to low-end as well as high-end users. Then make the site active instead of passive. Simply putting up a great site will benefit you, but if you work on drawing people to the site, you'll have more visitors and more return visits. How can you make a passive site active? Post the URL everywhere you can. Negotiate with related sites to link to the site. Give people reasons to visit you. Update the site regularly and keep it fresh. Make live data available on the site. Include contact links and information-gathering forms. Staff should include a hot link to the site in their e-mail signatures. In addition to the Web site, the Internet offers communication avenues such as electronic newsletters (your own and others on request), bulk e-mail, and perhaps paid advertising or paid postings and linkings.

17. *What about paying for Web advertising? What's available and what works?*

17. Most of us use Web search engines to find what we want. Knowing this, we should realize that the more often a site comes up in Web searches, the more visitors we will have at the site. Bringing about this search engine visibility has become big business. As search engines become more sophisticated in selecting relevant sites and pages, organizations have begun to hire people to work on "Web optimization." There are simple things you can do on your own using meta-tags and accurate titles, but I suggest talking to an expert about maximizing search engine visibility.

As for paid ads, like banners and sidebars, they're expensive and responses will be hard to track. If you choose paid Web advertising, be very sure you're reaching the specific market, and build in a tracking mechanism you can be confident about.

18. *How do we reassure customers about the security of our site?*

18. Again, institutional affiliation will reassure people that they can trust you. But beyond that, include a very visible privacy statement. Assure site visitors that information they leave with you will stay with you. Tell them how you will and will *not* use their information. If you want to develop a privacy statement, you can find many samples at sites doing a lot of e-commerce.

19. *We know people look for a sense of community. Is that possible on the Web?*

19. We have good research to support learning cohorts. When e-learners start a course together, collaborate, and get to know each other, they're more likely to complete the course and speak positively about their experience. There are others things organizations can do to provide a personal touch for the distance student: establish opt-in e-mail newsletters; provide friendly, efficient student services; celebrate students' successes by publishing graduation notices and personal profiles; and help them get to know and appreciate their instructors by including bios and photos in print and electronic publications.

20. *What are the two keys to success in marketing?*

20. Customer-focused research and planning.

RESOURCES

Dyché, J. (2001). *The CRM handbook: A business guide to customer relationship management.* Boston: Addison-Wesley Information Technology Series.

Allen, C., Kania, D., & Yaekel, B. (1998). *Internet world guide to one-to-one Web marketing.* New York: Wiley Computer Publishing.

Peppers, D., & Rogers, M. (1993). *The one to one future: Building relationships one customer at a time.* New York: Currency Doubleday.

Section 3:
E-Learning Tools and Platforms

Who would have thought that healthcare educators would be talking about "platforms," "learning management systems," "Web design tools," "discussion boards," "font size," or "servers"? These are the "tools of the trade" for e-learning course development, and being able to use them is becoming one of the new core competencies for educators. Should you purchase or lease these tools and platforms? Should you work with a company who will manage them for you? If you are confused about these terms and where to turn, the experts who have written the chapters in this unit will clarify them for you. In spite of the need to talk about the technology tools and platforms, it is important to keep learners in the forefront, use your knowledge of pedagogical principles, and integrate your expertise into the online course. Thus, this unit ends with the educators' view— answers to your questions about how to get started using the tools and platforms of e-learning and why.

Chapter 8: *Learning Management Systems*

1. What is a Learning Management System?

1. Learning Management Systems are comprehensive, "all-in-one," software packages for the delivery and management of Web-based courses. They provide a home for the course and allow access for you and students. Learning management systems are often compared to Swiss army knives with a variety of tools in one package as they include a variety of communication and course management tools. There are many popular commercial vendors: Blackboard, Convene, e-College, Embanet, WBT Systems, and WebCT are but a few.

2. How do learning management systems help with an online course?

2. Rather than building a custom site for a course, you are provided with tools that are relatively easy to learn. You do not have to focus on developing the technology, but rather on developing the course. These systems do not require much technical know-how. If you don't have the technical expertise, these ready-made options would be desirable.

3. What are the components or tools?

3. There are many features, but the core features have to do with student management and tracking, presentation of materials, communications, scheduling, and testing of students. Although there are no standards, student profiles, gradebooks, and online help are often included. These systems usually put an emphasis on collaboration with discussion forums and areas for student projects.

4. What are student management tools?

4. Students are provided with login and passwords into the course. A student roster is compiled and can be maintained to allow for limited access to the course. This protects the confidentiality of the course communications.

5. What is student tracking?

5. When students log into a course the tracking software records the time of the log in and the length of time spent in the course. The number of messages read and posted to forums or bulletin boards may also be recorded. This allows an educator to keep track of student activity. Some learners may not be entering the course and others may be "lurking" or only reading messages and not responding to others. This allows you to quickly gauge levels of participation.

6. What are bulletin boards or discussion forums?

6. This is usually the most important tool in Web-based courses. This form of communication allows you to create a community of learning through discussions. The terms bulletin boards and forums are used interchangeably to designate spaces for posting messages. The postings are like e-mail messages, except they are posted for the rest of the class to see. They are like letters in the mail. They can be read and responded to at any time; they are asynchronous communications.

7. What is a threaded message?

7. Messages in a bulletin board or a discussion forum may be related. This is called a conversation thread or message thread. This allows you to easily follow the dialogue on a topic. Threaded messages may be indented or some other indicator may be used to indicate that there are replying messages. The first message and replies (replies to replies) taken together is called a "message thread." It is very important in Web-based discussions to follow threads and post messages in the proper place.

8. Is there course mail or course e-mail?

8. This form of private electronic message communication is available within learning management systems. Messages can be sent to individuals or multiple recipients. An attachment feature is often useful for sending papers or other assignments.

9. What are attachments?

9. The sending and exchange of files can be done through an attachment feature, which allows you to send files through e-mail or sometimes in discussion forums. The person receiving or downloading the file must have the same software that created the file on his/her computer for the file to open. Thus, software standards are needed in Web-based courses to ensure the exchange of files.

10. What are chats?

10. The chat tool is useful for synchronous communication (communicating with someone at the same time). Chats are analogous to the telephone. The number of participants in a chat can vary from two to many. Chats are not threaded and keeping track of the conversation can be difficult with many participants. Chats can give a sense of immediacy and presence to a Web-based course, but they are difficult to schedule and conduct. Chat tools are useful for learning activities that require consensus building or for the quick resolution of a problem.

11. *What are whiteboards?*

11. This is a graphical electronic conferencing system for the simultaneous transmission of images such as a diagram, flow chart, or any other image that can be drawn usually with a mouse or a stylus.

12. *How are templates used?*

12. Templates allow you to standardize the look of Web pages. Preset headings, font types and sizes, colors, and white space will allow you to keep a clean and consistent look to the pages you use to deliver content. This allows you to quickly develop pages and ensures uniformity of presentations.

13. *How do I include pictures and graphics?*

13. Since we are operating in a Web environment, pictures or photographs must be in JPEG (Joint Photographic Experts Group) format. This format allows for smaller file size pictures that can be delivered on the Web. Line or simple drawings, as used in logos, are usually GIF (Graphic Interchange Format) files.

14. *What are learning objects?*

14. In Web-based courses it is better to think in small units. These small units are called learning objects. They are like building blocks that can be arranged to create a structure. Learning objects can be bought, sold, or traded. This allows you to customize a course as to topics or to quickly meet the needs of different students. This facilitates the easy editing and compilation of lessons and courses. For examples, look at the Merlot site: **http://www.merlot.org/Home.po**

15. *What are student pages and profiles?*

15. Student pages and profiles are a space for students or learners to create a "homepage" with their pictures and information relating their experience or hobbies. This allows students to get to know and get a "picture" of each other. This feature of learning management systems is important when creating a learning community.

16. *What are portfolios?*

16. Portfolios are a space for student to store information, their work, and projects. Students may share their project or submit them for grading in a portfolio space. This space is an electronic repository for storing and collecting students' work.

17. *How are tests provided?*

17. Traditional multiple choice, true/false, and matching exams are easily provided online from test banks. The questions are often presented in a random fashion and are immediately scored, with students given feedback. A time limit can often be set or the student may be allowed to take the exam multiple times for mastery.

Other varieties of exams, such as short answer or essay tests, are often provided in the exam tools. Course evaluations can be conducted in a similar fashion as exams.

18. What are gradebooks?

18. In an electronic version of the traditional gradebook, grades are recorded and shared online. Grades can be often automatically calculated and immediately distributed to students. Many gradebooks can import and export files such as spreadsheets, thus, simplifying grades.

19. Do I need all of these tools?

19. You can select the tools that fit a particular course. If there are some tools that are not needed, usually they can be hidden from the students' view. This allows you to pick and choose what is appropriate for the course.

20. What are benefits of a learning management system?

20. If you are pressed for time to develop a course or if your technical expertise is limited, a learning management system may be for you. If you are comfortable with the operation of a personal computer, it is relatively easy to learn to use these systems. Learning management systems bring a variety of tools into one integrated environment.

21. What are the disadvantages of a learning management system?

21. Advanced users often feel constrained by the tools and the configuration of the system.

22. What is more important, the technology or the pedagogy?

22. Although the technology is always a concern, there is usually a way to do what you want. The pedagogy of Web-courses is centered on collaborative learning and helping students construct their knowledge. The technology should be transparent or easy to use.

23. How do I manage a course?

23. The good news is that the class is always available. The bad news is the class is always available. Time management and self-directed learning are primary in Web-based courses. You will have to set limits on your participation and the amount of time devoted to attending to the course. Otherwise, you feel that you are always in class.

24. Where do I go for help?

24. When selecting a learning management system, you should evaluate the services provided to the users by the company. Service should be a prime consideration in the evaluation when purchasing the system. Determine

25. Can I do this myself?

25. Developing a Web-based course is often a team effort. You may need assistance with instructional development, Web page design, programming, copyright clearance, and even graphic design.

26. Where do I go from here?

the level of local support for the technology and the learning management software.

26. After selecting learning management software, the real works begins of developing, designing, implementing, and evaluating a course. Developing Web-based courses involves a lot of up-front work before the course is ready to use.

RESOURCES

Hall, B. (1997). *Web-based training.* New York: John Wiley & Sons.

Kahn, B. H. (Ed.). (1997). *Web-based instruction.* Englewood Cliffs, NJ: Educational Technology Publications.

McCormack, C., & Jones, D. (1997). *Building a web-based education system.* New York: John Wiley & Sons.

Palloff, R. M., & Pratt, K. (1999). *Building learning communities in cyberspace.* San Francisco: Jossey-Bass, Inc.

Blackboard—**http://www.blackboard.com**

Learning Spaces—**http://www.lotus.com**

TopClass—**http://www.wbtsystems.com**

Virtual-U—**http://www.vlei.com/**

WebCT—**http://www.webct.com**

Chapter 9: *Advanced Tools: Video and Audio*

1. *What is digital audio?*

1. Audio is recorded as a digital file so that it can be played on computer. In the past, audiotape recorders used continuous or analog signals on tape. There are many audio formats, including aiff (Apple Instrument File Format), which was developed for the Macintosh computer; .wav (wave) is the standard for Windows; and MPEG-MP3 is currently popular, which is compressed to reduce file size. Compression reduces the parts of the sound that are irrelevant to the reproduction of the sound. This is the technology that allows the file size to be smaller. MIDI (Musical Instrument Digital Interface) provides a means for synchronizing electronic musical instruments. Streaming audio, like streaming video, is a popular file format used on the Web. You don't have to wait to download the sound files. The files begin playing (streaming) while still downloading. Experts consider the sound quality on the Web to be good.

2. *How would audio files be used in a class?*

2. Audio files are often used as an alert or to gain attention in the computer environment.

Lectures can be recorded and used with PowerPoint with audio, which can be downloaded from the Web. Remember that five minutes in the Web environment is a long time. A welcome message with your picture would be a good way to introduce yourself to the class. This personalizes the message and reinforces your presence.

3. *What is video and audio streaming?*

3. Rather than waiting to download the files, which can take a long time from minutes to hours, video and audio are played as files are downloaded. Streaming is like a faucet that is turned on, when drips of water become a stream.

4. *What is digital video?*

4. Digital video refers to video images that can be recognized by a computer. QuickTime, Windows Media, and Real Media formats are used on the Web. Video files are extremely large. Five minutes of uncompressed video would use about one gigabyte of space. Compression looks for similarities within and between frames to reduce the size of the video file. You need to consider the data rate, frame rate, and the window size you will use for distribution. Streaming video allows you to start playing (streaming) video before it is downloaded. Most students will not have significant bandwidth at home to view video clips. Videos may appear jerky and choppy to those using slower modem speeds or due to network traffic. At this time, experts consider the quality of video on the Web to be poor.

5. What equipment do I need to create digital video?

5. You can use a digital camera with a firewire connection to your computer or a video capture card to transfer the video from a standard VHS tape or camera. You will need software to edit and compress the video for distribution on the Web. There are many software programs from which to choose. Adobe Premiere is often the software selected to do both of these procedures.

6. What software is needed to play videos on the Web?

6. Three major formats for users are QuickTime, developed for Macintosh platform, Windows Media, and Real Media Player. The video must be encoded for the each of the formats. Real Media uses a special server for the video and streaming is done in real-time. Windows Media is progressive streaming (on demand) and downloads it to your hard drive. Real-time streaming is usually broadcast directly to a browser from a special server. Progressive streaming is probably the easier route for beginners to use, as no special server equipment is required.

7. Why is video compression needed before you distribute?

7. Even if the video is in digital form, you still need another step before it can be easily used on the Web. The file size needs to set for a 28.8 modem, with a data rate of 2.5 KB per second. DVD players have a data rate of 1 MB per second. Smaller files require lower data transfer rates, enabling smooth video playback. So, it's important to match file size to data rate of the intended machine.

8. Can I use videos that I use in class on the Web?

8. You first must get copyright clearance to do this and this isn't always easy to do. Remember that the quality of the video depends upon the bandwidth available to the end users. Most videos would need to be broken down into small segments or clips. A summary in textual form should be available as a back up in case the students have problems with the clips.

9. What is the best use of video in Web-based courses?

9. Video is very effective for demonstrations or where motion is important to learning. Video is a powerful representation of reality and can be used to personalize the course.

A short introduction of yourself and to the course is an ideal use. Remember that shorter is better on the Web. Aim for three-minute clips. Windows-based video e-mail is a good way to give students personalized feedback.

10. What about using PowerPoint in my courses?

10. Microsoft PowerPoint 2000 has a feature called Presentation Broadcast that allows for the synchronizing of PowerPoint images with live or recorded presentations. A number of new software programs make it easy to combine PowerPoint with audio narration to create streaming presentations. Audio streaming with slides produces good quality sound and effective presentations.

11. What is the future of video streaming?

11. Streaming is the future for Web technology. As bandwidth increases and converges with other trends, like increased computing power, and the proliferation of the Web itself, interactive video streaming will be a critical opportunity for Web-based learning.

When streaming video is used in Web pages, the presentation may include embedded links for further information. Streaming content can be used to trigger other Web page events, such as graphics, animations, or links to other pages. These multiple points of access will take streaming video beyond the linear narrative.

RESOURCES

Jakob Nielsen's Alertbox, August 8, 1999—**http://www.useit.com/alertbox/990808.html**

RealPlayer—**http://www.real.com/**

Streaming Media World: Video Tutorial—**http://www.streamingmediaworld.com/video/tutor/**

Webmonkey: Streaming Audio Tutorial—**http://hotwired.lycos.com/webmonkey/00/45/ index3a.html?tw=multimedia**

Webmonkey: Streaming Video—**http://hotwired.lycos.com/webmonkey/geektalk/97/10/ index4a.html?tw=multimedia**

Webmonkey: Streaming Video for the Masses—**http://hotwired.lycos.com/webmonkey/01/03/ index4a.html?tw=multimedia**

Windows Media Player—**http://windowsmedia.com/download/download.asp**

Chapter 10: Options for Choosing and Using Course Development and Management Tools

1. What kinds of tools are available to develop and manage e-learning?

1. There are as many different tools for developing and managing e-learning as there are ways to deliver instruction online. The tools you choose to make up an e-learning system will depend on the approach you take—will you build your own system from scratch, purchase multiple products to meet various needs, or purchase an all-in-one solution? If you decide to "do-it-yourself," you will need to look into development tools, including programming languages, authoring programs, and application software for developing course content and collaboration tools yourself, or with the help of a team of developers. If you take the second approach, to "piece-it-together," you will need to investigate ready-made tools that can be purchased, each of which is tailored to perform a single e-learning function within a course. These components can be pieced together to provide the specific functionality you need for an online course. In many cases, you may find that the best approach is to purchase an "all-in-one" solution, which provides in one package all or most of the tools you need for e-learning. The approach you decide to take will depend on the availability of technical resources, your budget, and your timeline for implementing a solution.

2. How do I know which tools to choose?

2. During the early implementation of e-learning, the type of content that made up most e-learning courses consisted mainly of simple Web pages with little interaction. Simple development tools, such as an IITML editor or even a word processing program, sufficed to get the job done. As e-learning courses increasingly take advantage of advanced interactive features, such as message forums, chats, and even video conferencing, the software and skills needed to develop these tools increases exponentially. For all but the simplest e-learning content, you will probably not want to develop your own solution from scratch, unless you need customized solutions that can't be purchased off the shelf, and you have a team of developers to assist in the creation of these tools.

3. Is it better to purchase an all-in-one product or to piece together components?

3. Piecing together an e-learning platform with specialized components gives you more flexibility to tailor tools to your needs. However, making the components work together can be a technical challenge. Imagine, for example, that you purchase a message forum tool from

one vendor and a chat program from another. Each tool has its own database of student accounts. Will you have to create an account for each student for each tool? Will students have to log in to each tool separately? If the tools have been developed following emerging standards, then the integration should be possible. Regardless, making the integration happen can still be a technical challenge. Even if the integration of the components is doable, students might find switching from one tool to another to be confusing if the user interface for each tool is substantially different.

An "all-in-one" product eliminates many of the complexities of implementing various components, but it usually suffers from not being able to provide the same level of functionality. It is a tremendous advantage and a potential cost savings, however, to be able to work with a single vendor rather than multiple vendors of specialized tools.

A decision about which strategy to pursue will depend on a careful assessment of the type of functionality you need in an e-learning system (see Table 1).

Table 1. *Three Approaches to Implementing an E-Learning System*

	Advantages	Disadvantages
Do-It-Yourself	Allows for maximum customization of the learning product	Requires advanced development skills Very time-consuming to develop solutions
Piece-It-Together	Takes advantage of the best tools available for specific learning objectives Can add and remove components as needed to achieve an optimal blend of tools for your needs	Can be difficult to integrate various components into a seamless solution More difficult to implement than an all-in-one solution
All-In-One	Relatively fast and easy to implement Well-integrated toolset	Integrated tools often lack advanced functionality Can be difficult to customize

4. Why are IMS and other standards important?

4. Instructional Management Systems (IMS), now the IMS Global Learning Consortium, Inc., is a global consortium with members from educational, commercial, and government organizations that is developing specifications for facilitating online distributed learning activities such as locating and using educational content, tracking learner progress, reporting learner performance, and exchanging student records between administrative systems. The importance of this and other standards, such as the Sharable Content Object Reference Model (SCORM™) and the Aviation Industry CBT (Computer-Based Training) Committee (AICC), is to help ensure that products that you may purchase can "talk" to each other. This helps not only to facilitate easy integration of various products into a seamless e-learning system, but also ensures that content you create in one system can be easily transferred to another system.

The importance of these standards should be obvious if you are attempting to piece together components from various manufacturers into an e-learning system. But even if you decide on an all-in-one solution you need to be mindful of an all-in-one product's adherence to standards. Imagine that you develop several e-learning courses in an all-in-one product, and the vendor goes out of business. If the product represents the content of the course in a proprietary way, you may be unable to easily transfer the content to a new system.

5. What are some available tools if I decide to piece together an e-learning system?

5. The number of available e-learning tools is large and constantly changing. Table 2 provides a categorized list of a small set of these tools. For more information on these and other tools, see:
http://www.osc.edu/education/webed/

Table 2. **E-Learning Tools**

Discussion Tools

Allaire Forums http://www.allaire.com/Products/forums/	Now an open source product after Allaire merger with Macromedia
NiceNet http://www.nicenet.org/	Free conferencing service
Discus http://www.discusware.com/	Basic version is free

continued on page 70

Table 2, continued from page 69

Conferencing Tools (chat, video conferencing)

Centra Conference and Symposium http://www.centra.com/	Conferencing software and a virtual classroom with audio and video capabilities
CUSeeMe Conference Server http://www.cuseeme.com/	Software-only video conferencing software
HorizonLive http://www.horizonlive.com/	Virtual classroom software
LearnLinc http://www.mentergy.com/	Virtual classroom software
NetMeeting http://www.microsoft.com/netmeeting/	Free video conferencing software. Allows only one-to-one audio and video conferencing

Testing Tools

Exam Builder http://www.exambuilder.com/	An online service for creating exams
Question Mark Perception http://www.questionmark.com/	Online assessment tool

Development Tools

Macromedia's Authorware and Director www.macromedia.com	Advanced multimedia authoring software
Macromedia's Flash www.macromedia.com	Authoring software for creating animations
Hot Potatoes http://web.uvic.ca/hrd/halfbaked/	Software to easily create interactive multiple-choice, short-answer, jumbled-sentence, crossword, matching/ordering, and gap-fill exercises
Toolbook II Assistant and Instructor http://www.click2learn.com/	Advanced multimedia authoring software

6. What are some popular "all-in-one" products?

6. Table 3 lists a small set of available all-in-one products. There are many such products targeted to businesses that are not included here.

Table 3. **All-In-One Products**

Blackboard http://www.blackboard.com	Easy-to-use software. Offers free course creation on their servers
ClassPoint http://www.cuseeme.com/	Incorporates advanced video conferencing capabilities
LearningSpace http://www.lotus.com/learningspace	IBM software, well integrated with Lotus Notes
TopClass http://www.wbtsystems.com/	Good content management. Allows for customized paths through the content
Virtual-U http://www.vlei.com/	Very customizable. Includes source code for advanced customization
WebCT http://www.webct.com	Good customization and student tracking features

7. What criteria should I use to assess the quality of available tools?

7. I recommend talking to people in other areas of the organization who may already have experience with available tools, and getting in touch with other organizations similar to your own that have already implemented e-learning systems. Since there are so many available tools, this will help you focus attention on some of the more popular tools used widely by organizations similar to your own. There are also many resources on the Web that provide detailed comparisons of products and vendors, such as: **http://www.c2t2.ca/landon-line/**

Some of the more important factors you will want to consider when evaluating products include:

- Be sure that the product supports the features you are looking for and that the cost is within your budget.

- The product should be tested for ease-of-use, both for students and instructors. You may want to sacrifice some advanced features in favor of ease-of-use.

- You will want to work with the technology manager in your organization to be sure that you have the resources to meet the product's hardware and software requirements, as well as to be sure the organization has the personnel with the skills and time to install and maintain the product.

- Ensure that the product meets accessibility, privacy, security, and other regulatory requirements of the organization.

- Test the product to be sure that all potential client programs (usually Web browsers—Netscape/Internet Explorer) work with the program.

- Assess how well the vendor is able to support the product.

8. Does the popularity of a particular product make it a more viable solution?

8. The popularity of an e-learning product might be an important consideration when shopping for a solution. As instructors increasingly push to stretch current technology to provide more enriching e-learning experiences for students, it is becoming increasingly more expensive to produce more interactive content for courses. Most organizations cannot afford to support this high level of development for all but a few courses. The solution to this is to purchase off-the-shelf "modules" of highly interactive content that can be plugged into your e-learning system. This might also be done for simple content for which the organization has no in-house content expert. Many textbook publishers, for example, are providing multimedia content and electronic test question banks with their textbooks. Publishers, who are able to provide this content at a reasonable cost by targeting large markets, are likely only to provide this content in a format that plugs easily into the most popular e-learning products. If you use less popular e-learning products, or if you develop a proprietary e-learning system within the organization, you may find that you are unable to integrate off-the-shelf content into your e-learning system.

As product vendors begin to adopt standards, such as IMS, for representing content, this will afford organizations more flexibility in the products they choose. Publishers will begin to package content in compliance with open standards rather than to work with proprietary systems.

9. Is it better to manage our own servers or to pay a hosting service?

9. As you investigate what products will meet e-learning needs, you need to determine if you have the hardware, software (operating systems), technical personnel, and the network bandwidth to support the e-learning system. This should only be done in collaboration with the director of technical operations for your organization. If you do have the necessary resources, hosting an e-learning system internally can be cost-effective, and will afford the flexibility to adapt to changing needs quickly. If, however, your internal technical resources are not adequate, you may want to consider outsourcing your e-learning system to a hosting service.

Outsourcing an e-learning system can also be cost-effective, depending on the scale of your plans. The marketplace for hosting companies is somewhat volatile, so you do run the risk of jeopardizing the continuity of e-learning operations if the hosting company closes or merges.

10. Who offers e-learning hosting?

10. Table 4 lists a few of the companies that offer e-learning hosting.

Table 4. *A Sampling of E-Learning Hosting Providers*

Blackboard	http://www.blackboard.com
CollegisEduprise, Inc.	http://www.collegiseduprise.com
Convene	http://www.convene.com/
eCollege	http://www.ecollege.com/
Digital Learning Interactive (iLrn)	http://www.digitlearn.org
Education To Go	http://www.educationtogo.com/
eWebUniversity	http://www.ewebuniversity.com
Jones Knowledge	http://www.jonesknowledge.com/
MetaCollege	http://metacollege.com/
VCampus	http://www.vcampus.com/webuol/

11. What kind of servers do we need?

11. Assuming that you decide to host the e-learning system internally, you will need to purchase a server (or more than one depending on your set of products and anticipated student numbers). You may be able to take advantage of existing servers in the organization. You should discuss the available server resources with the manager of your organization's technical resources. If you find that you will need to purchase a server, you can expect to spend anywhere from $5,000 to $30,000 or more, depending on your specific needs. Besides the server, you will need to ensure that you have purchased additional hardware and software to support reliable backups and security, and be sure that you have well-trained technical staff to care for the servers.

12. What skills are needed to develop custom e-learning solutions?

12. If you decide to venture down the path of building a custom e-learning solution from scratch, be sure that you have access to highly competent technical staff, depending on the complexity of the solution you are considering. Even a relatively simple task such as creating a Web page will require substantial technical assistance to set up a Web site, move the page to the Web site, and set the proper permissions on the page. Table 5 presents some typical e-learning development activities, and the skills needed to accomplish them.

Table 5. *Typical E-Learning Tools/Content, and Technical Skills Needed to Develop Them*

Tool or Content	Needed Skills
Creating simple Web pages	Ability to use an HTML editor, word processing program, presentation software, or other application software to create Web pages.
Creating Web graphics	Ability to use an illustration program or photo editing software. Familiarity with .jpg and .gif graphic formats, screen resolutions, color palettes, pixel dimensions, and other computer graphics concepts.
Creating animations	Ability to use an authoring program (such as Macromedia Flash or Director) or programming language (such as Java). Familiarity with programming concepts and multimedia design.

continued on page 75

Table 5, continued from page 74

Tool or Content	Needed Skills
Incorporating audio and video	Ability to use video editing hardware and software. Familiarity with video codes and streaming technologies.
Creating course management tools (e.g., testing tools, message forum tools, chat tools)	Strong programming experience. Familiarity with multi-tier (or client/server) application design and previous Web application design experience.

13. *Can I purchase subject-specific content or courses "off the shelf" for use in a course?*

13. Depending on what content you are looking for, you may be able to purchase subject-specific content to plug into the course, or perhaps even purchase an entire course for delivery in an organization. You are more likely to find such content if the subject has a wide audience. A good place to start looking for this content is to contact the publishers of textbooks in the subject you are interested in.

14. *What are the costs involved in deploying an e-learning system?*

14. The cost of deploying an e-learning system will vary tremendously depending on existing resources, the products you choose to use, and the hardware and software that will be needed to support the products you choose. As you plan deployment, keep in mind that the plan will need to be flexible to account for changes and additions as needed, and should incorporate a life-cycle replacement plan for computer hardware and software upgrades. Table 6 illustrates a fictitious deployment scenario with estimated costs, which should give you an idea of some of the costs involved.

Table 6. *Sample E-Learning Deployment Cost Sheet*

Item	Cost	Cost Per Year
Server (including operating system software, backup hardware/software/media, and other management and security software)	$20,000	$5,000 (assuming a 4 year life-cycle)
All-in-one course management system	$5,000	$5,000
Technical personnel (50% time of system administrator to manage server and software)	$25,000	$25,000
TOTAL	$50,000	$35,000

RESOURCES

Distance learning tools: A guide to online tools and services for teaching and learning at a distance [Entire issue]. (2000). *Syllabus, 13*(10).

Randy, B. (1999). *Educational technology planning*. Victoria, BC, Canada: Centre for Curriculum, Transfer, & Technology.

Chapter 11: Getting Started With E-Learning Tools and Platforms: An Educator's View

1. When did you get started?

1. I have been privileged to use technology in my teaching since 1998, and I continue to be in awe of its great power and endless possibilities. I work hard in my role as a nurse educator, and for me, creating e-learning environments for students has been most enjoyable and worthwhile work. I take my work very seriously, and because I believe that the end product of my work is student learning, I take great pride in all that my students have been able to learn, assisted by the use of instructional technology.

2. How do you feel about e-learning?

2. While I take my work very seriously, at the same time, I tend to take the technology rather lightly. From the very beginning, my level of enthusiasm for the use of instructional technology has always been far greater than my level of technological expertise. Fortunately, the quantity, quality, and availability of e-learning tools has grown rapidly over the past few years. If you know what it is you would like to do, chances are there is already an e-learning tool available to help you do it well. Now, more than ever before, e-learning tools are becoming better and easier to use.

3. What has changed over the past few years?

3. Today, we are more aware of the need to design online course components based on the content and not based on the technology. We are also better able to see that the true benefits of e-learning are not related to the instructional technology itself. The success of e-learning is directly related to the use of tried and true pedagogy and the teaching methods that the instructional technology supports.

4. How did you get started?

4. I teach beginning students in an undergraduate program who most often are not aware of the general rule of thumb that for every contact hour in the classroom, there are also an expected three associated study hours apart from classroom learning. Students spend one third of their learning time in the classroom, and two thirds of their learning time alone, on their own, outside of class. I wanted to find ways to support that two thirds of student learning taking place outside of the classroom.

5. What was the best thing that happened once you started?

5. While trying to create opportunities for students to become more active learners, I became a more active teacher! I found myself more connected to the learners and that the learning was not constrained by place, time,

learning speed, or learning style. What a wonderful surprise! Not only did the students become more actively engaged, but so did I.

6. Why should I want to do this?

6. Teaching on the Web is a way for you to improve what you teach, how you teach, and most important, how students learn. You will become less focused on "teaching students" and more focused on "students learning." You will come to see yourself as a guide, motivator, and coach, whose focus is on content and time on task. You will have worldwide resources. You will enjoy the challenge of using technology to help students learn. You will marvel at how easily you accomplish course management activities.

7. How much time is it going to take?

7. First, remember that no matter where it happens, good teaching is good teaching, and good teaching is hard work! At first, it may seem to take more time to develop e-learning components. But, later on you may find that there is no significant amount of difference in preparation time as compared to preparation time for traditional courses. While you are spending more time on some things, you are spending less time on others. Eventually, you may come to feel that any additional time devoted to e-learning is enjoyable time well spent, and wonder how you could ever teach again without using instructional technology.

8. How do I get started?

8. The very best way to get started is to spend some time reflecting on *what* it is you want to do, rather than *how* will you do it. What do you want to accomplish with e-learning tools and platforms? Remind yourself that most of us are reluctant to change the familiar ways we do things, but that it is easy to get used to a new way of doing things if that new way is also a better way. Hang on to your traditionally sound pedagogy, and take it with you as you go online. At the same time, surrender yourself to a new, better way of doing what it is that you already do. Give up, give in, let go, don't fight it! When starting, it is far more important to be willing than it is to be able.

9. What is the easiest part about getting started?

9. The most important component of e-learning is the *content*, which you probably already have. If you are a good teacher in the classroom, you will become an even better teacher by using instructional technology. If you really like teaching in the classroom, you will love teaching online. You and the learners will be able to interact with the subject matter like never before. Technology itself does not improve student learning. You enhance student learning by using technology as a tool to create rich learning experiences.

10. What resources do I need to offer Web courses?

10. You already have the most important things you will need: the program outcomes, course competencies, and the course description. If you are already teaching these courses in a traditional classroom setting, you also have the syllabus, schedule of weekly classes, assignments, lectures, in class group learning activities, quizzes, exams, handouts, grade book, and so on. All of these can be easily converted to an online course.

11. What other resources do I need?

11. Find and use something called learning management software, or "courseware," a Web-based program that will allow you to author and manage your course. It could be that your institution has developed a "house brand," or you might consider others. Many listed in Table 1 provide sample and demonstration courses. Some will allow you to try their course software free for a limited time (see also Chapters 8, 9, 10).

Table 1. *Learning Management Software*

Asymetrix Learning System http://www.gy.com/company/asymet_ad.htm	Ecollege http://www.ecollege.com/company/
Avilar WebMentor http://www.avilar.com/	Eduprise http://www.eduprise.com/
Blackboard http://blackboard.com/	FlexTraining http://www.flextraining.com
Convene http://www.convene.com/	IntraKal http://www.anlon.com
ClassNet http://classnet.cc.iastate.edu/	Lotus LearningSpace http://www.lotus.com/home.nsf/ welcome/learnspace
CyberClass http://www.einstruction.com/ frmain01.htm	ClassWise http://www.classwise.com/
CyberProf http://www.howhy.com/home/obtaining/ obtaining.html	WebCT http://Webct.com/

12. *Which course authoring/ management software do you think is the best?*

12. I think that they are all good in one way or another. While none of them are perfect, it is easier to use existing software than to try to create it yourself.

13. *What course authoring/ management software do you use?*

13. From the start, I have chosen to use the courseware developed by my institution. By using the in-house software, I believe that I am supporting the work of the developers. User feedback provides the developers with important information they need to make the product better. If you hear that there are "problems" with your institution's software, use it anyway and find out for yourself. Let the developers know what works and what could be made better. Be part of the solution!

14. *Who will give me encouragement to do this work?*

14. Your greatest source of encouragement will come from students. While students are quick to let you know what they don't like, they are often slow to give positive feedback. Imagine how you will feel when, without even asking, you get positive comments about e-learning from students! Many times they will let you know what they want and what they need. Often these are things you haven't thought of. It is easier to believe in yourself after others have believed in you first.

15. *What do students say they like best about e-learning?*

15. Students like those things that are interactive. They want to do more than just "view and print." They also like those things that are useful to them, things that save them time, and things that make learning easier. They also like knowing that all their course materials reside on the Web, and are as near to them as any Web browser, on any computer, anywhere, and at anytime.

16. *What are some of the things I can do with a learning management system that works well?*

16.
- Syllabus
  - Students like an online syllabus because it never gets lost; it's always there on the Web.
  - Students like many active hyperlinks that they can click on for more information.
    - If you refer to a library make the word "library" a hyperlink that will take them to the library's Web site.
    - If you provide your e-mail address, create a hyperlink that will allow them to send mail by clicking on your e-mail address.
    - When you list the required texts, create

hyperlinks to the campus book store, or the publisher's textbook companion site.

+ If you refer to off campus meeting sites, include a hyperlink to a map with directions.

+ Make it usable and functional.

- Students sometimes like to use the course syllabus as a start page where they can go to "click through" to other Web pages.

• Schedule of Weekly Classes

- Many students use this as their "to do list." They like to know about weekly class content, weekly assignments, and what is due when.

- Here they like to find guidelines, instructions, and the rationale for learning activities.

- Chapter outlines, PowerPoint slides, and handouts can be downloaded and printed. Students often bring these to class to facilitate note taking.

- They can easily find resources you have selected to supplement their textbook learning.

- Other student favorites are charts, tables, forms, checklists, and templates that can be downloaded and used in word processors.

• Announcements

- Students prefer to find important messages on an announcement page rather than in an e-mail message.

- They like to look in one place to see if something has been added or has changed.

• Class Roster

- Students like creating their personal profile.

- They like reading other students' profiles.

- Pictures help them learn each other's names.

• E-mail

- Students like to click on a name to send a message with no need to know the address.

- They like being able to easily send a message to one student, several students, or the entire class.

- Students do not want to read a lot of e-mail and complain if they do.

- When given a choice they prefer to submit written assignments as courseware e-mail attachments.

- Discussion Forums

  - Students often find threaded discussion assignments to be tedious work.

  - They seldom voluntarily use discussion forums.

  - They will use discussion forums for getting needed answers if you:

    ◆ Create a discussion forum for each assignment.

    ◆ Instruct students to post assignment related questions there.

    ◆ Are slow to answer student questions. Other students will come to the rescue and answer the questions. They will learn from one another.

    ◆ Thank students for posting questions; thank students for answering questions.

    ◆ Give feedback about content and the learning process.

    ◆ Add missing points; correct misinformation.

    ◆ Stimulate discussion in higher levels of cognitive and affective domains.

- Chat Rooms

  - Very few students will participate in instructor chat sessions.

  - They are loathe to be one of the few present in the chat room with you.

  - They will use the chat room for group work if you:

    ◆ Create a chat room for each group of students working together on a presentation or project.

    ◆ Let the students know that the chat session will be archived.

    ◆ Create a chat room for students' private and social conversation.

- Tests and Surveys

  - Students like taking online practice quizzes if you:

    ◆ Allow students to see their score immediately upon completion.

- ◆ Provide the correct responses with rationale.
- ◆ Allow students unlimited time to complete the quiz.
- ◆ Allow students to take the quiz more than once.

  - Students enjoy completing self-assessment questionnaires online if you:
    - ◆ Provide directions for completing the self-assessment
    - ◆ Provide instructions for scoring and interpreting the results
    - ◆ Have students submit a summary of their findings.

  - Students prefer not to complete course and faculty evaluations online, because they believe that they will not be anonymous. If you do conduct course and faculty evaluations online, explain to the students how you are providing for anonymity (usually a function of the test and survey tool).

  - Students find online examinations to be stressful; their greatest fear is of losing their online connection.

- Gradebook

  - Students like being able to see their grades in a private online gradebook.

  - Students like receiving assignment grades and instructors' comments sooner.

- Online Tools and Resources

  - Students like being able to go to other Web sources without leaving the courseware e-learning environment

  - Provide students with links to all those Web resources you think will be useful.

- A "Getting Started" Assignment

  - Students should have an opportunity to work with e-learning tools early in the course. Here is an example used in the first lesson in a course for undergraduate students.

    - ◆ The purpose of this exercise is to ensure that you know how to use Oncourse (the learning management system). An understanding of the Oncourse environment is critical to your success in this class. The Oncourse tools we will be using in this course include e-mail with attachments, discussion forums, the gradebook, chat rooms, World Wide Web resources and iQuiz for review questions, practice quizzes, and self-assessments. Other tools we will be using include Microsoft Word, RealPlayer, and Internet Explorer. Some of you may already be familiar with these programs.

Complete the activities listed below:

◆ Write a short e-mail message that includes your full name, phone number, last four digits of your student ID, a little bit about yourself including your personal goals for this course. OR you may choose to create your message using Microsoft Word, save it to a file, and send the Word file you created as an Oncourse e-mail attachment.

◆ Go to the "My Profile" (homepage) section. Create your profile (homepage). If you have a picture or graphic you may upload it to your file manager and add the link to your profile. If you want, you may limit access to your profile information to faculty only. However, I recommend you allow fellow students to view your information as well. Remember, do not put anything in your profile you wouldn't want to be public.

◆ From the Oncourse Tools section visit the six netiquette Web sites listed under the section titled "Communicating on the Internet."

◆ Go to the Discussion Forum. Identify the site you liked the best and explain why; also identify the site you liked the least and why. Browse through the other messages in the forum to see what comments other students have posted. Post a reply to at least one student's message.

◆ Take Oncourse Practice Quiz One. (This is a "fun" quiz to acquaint the students with the testing tools.)

17. *What makes the best Web course to start with?*

17. I have found that the best course to start with is one that is Web-enhanced, rather than one that is totally Web-based. Focus on that two-thirds of student learning time that happens between classroom meetings. Use e-learning to complement classroom learning.

18. Where do I look for online learning resources?

18. Today, it is very common for publishers to provide an online companion Web-site to accompany student textbooks. These Web sites are rich with resources for students, and faculty as well. There you will find many e-teaching resources such as annotated chapter outlines and notes, PowerPoint presentations, transparency masters, images, test questions, suggested learning activities, and so forth. You will also find learning resources for students such as practice quizzes, games, Web links, and audio and video presentations, just to mention a few.

19. What worries do educators have about e-learning?

19. At first I worried about the technology. I just couldn't seem to believe that the courseware would do what it was supposed to do! For example, if I read and graded a student e-mail assignment, I couldn't trust that the grade would go from the e-mail section into the gradebook section and that a notification really would be sent to the student. I found myself double-checking things over and over, just to make sure things worked. I also worried that things would "disappear," and spent a lot of time printing copies of almost everything: the class roster, the gradebook, the assignments. I made back-up copies of my back-ups. Once I completed the first few weeks of the course, I found that it all really did work!

20. What final suggestions do you have for getting started?

20. I was one of the first persons on my campus to develop a Web course. Although I was able to figure out how to use the course management system by myself, I find that it is helpful to network with others who are also e-learning, and locating resources at a teaching support center. Each time I offer the course, I find I am adding new activities and resources to it.

RESOURCES

Boettcher, J. (1999). *Embracing Web learning: Faculty guide for moving courses to the Web.* **http://www.cren.net**

Collison, G., Elbaum, B., Jaavind, S., & Tinker, R. (2000). *Facilitating online learning.* Madison, WI: Atwood Publishing.

Harasim, L., Hiltz, R., Teles, L., & Taroff, M. (1997). *Learning networks: A field guide to teaching and learning online.* Cambridge, MA: MIT Press.

Palloff, R., & Pratt, K. (2001). *Lessons from the cyberspace classroom: The realities of online teaching.* San Francisco: Jossey-Bass.

Section 4:
E-Educators

The classroom has expanded beyond its four walls and is no longer the primary place for teaching and learning. Teaching in this new world—becoming an e-educator—requires taking risks, learning new skills, figuring out how to build relationships with students you may never see in person, grappling with your rights as an e-educator, managing your intellectual property, and finding new sources of satisfaction and rewards for your work. This can, at times, feel like you are moving from expert to novice. At the same time, becoming an e-educator is an opportunity to renew your commitment to learners, to make the shift from teaching to learning, and to redefine your role. Good news: your teaching skills are still intact, and once you are on the other side of the technology and course design learning curves, you are still grounded by your philosophy, values, and expertise. The authors in this unit give you a "heads up" about these changes, and share their strategies for making the transition to your role as an e-educator.

Chapter 12: How Do I Learn to Teach on the Web?

1. Where do I learn how to teach in online courses?

1. The first steps are to find resources to help you master the concepts of online learning. Will you have technical support or will you be doing this all on your own? This is very important as a beginner. Depending upon your level of comfort and the availability of support, you may want to look into courses offered through local technical/community colleges. Become comfortable with the basics of your computer and how to use the Web. If you feel really comfortable with using your computer and the Web, online courses allow you to apply knowledge as you learn Web course design.

2. What resources are available to educators to learn to teach Web courses?

2. A multitude of resources are available to instructors who are ready to teach on the Web. There are books, journals, Web sites, news groups, and listservs which focus on online teaching. One of the best resources is the U.S. Department of Education (DOE) Web site known as "Ask Eric" (**http://www.askeric.org/**). This Web site provides access to the DOE database. A recent search using the terms "online teaching" resulted in 75 references. Individuals can review an abstract for each reference and then obtain a full-text copy. Other online resources include the Google™ search engine (**www.google.com**) which uses a software robot called Googlebot to identify and evaluate more than a billion pages of content on the Web. This allows for a comprehensive search that can be based on a question such as "What resources are available to educators to learn to teach Web courses?" A recent Google search on the preceding question resulted in 195,000 hits in 0.45 seconds. The hits are listed in order of relevance, so the researcher can easily locate the most appropriate listing.

3. How does content in e-learning differ from classroom content?

3. Course content does not necessarily have to differ between a traditional course and an online course. The difference is in the delivery. While traditional course instructors may rely primarily on outside reading, lecture, discussion, and testing, an online course will require a different approach to student-to-instructor and student-to-student interaction. Content can be delivered in an online course as text based material (e.g., as an HTML page, a PDF file, a Word document), as an online slide presentation (e.g., PowerPoint), or in a threaded discussion group. Instructors can include graphics, video clips, material on CD ROMs, outside reading in

textbooks, journals, and online material as well. The challenge for instructors is how to convert their content to an online format. This requires a comprehensive faculty development program that gives instructors the skills and knowledge they need to successfully convert their content. In the absence of a faculty development program, individual instructors may need to independently develop the knowledge and skills using the resources mentioned here.

4. How much time does it take to teach using e-learning methods?

4. The amount of time needed to teach an online course varies depending on the level of interaction and the number of graded assignments. Courses that require students to complete reading assignments and take online exams with little interaction with the instructor will obviously require little time on the part of the instructor and would be considered a low maintenance course. However, courses that require students to post questions to a threaded discussion and/or respond to the instructor or other student postings, could require an instructor to log in to the course several times a week and spend one to two hours answering and/or responding to student questions/comments. Courses that require the electronic submission of weekly assignments will also require a substantial time commitment on the part of the instructor. It is important to note that once students become comfortable with online interaction, they will begin to communicate on a regular basis and expect the instructor to respond on a timely basis.

5. Will I need to learn about teaching on the Web all at once?

5. Learning to teach on the Web requires many new skills and methods to deliver content. The time required to learn and master these skills varies for each person, but learning the process in small steps makes mastery easier and more enjoyable. Start the first course small in both content and number of learners. As you master this, you need less time and can then expand your skills into new phases of online teaching. The learning curve to learn to teach on the Web is very big and will take time to master, so just be patient with yourself.

6. Will one hour of classroom teaching be the same if Web-based?

6. Because of the asynchronous nature of online courses, it is very difficult to equate one hour of classroom instruction to an equivalent time online. Online teaching requires instructors to move from a pedagogical approach to an androgogical approach to teaching. Students become much more involved in, and responsible for,

their learning. The instructor ensures that the content is available, but then acts more as a guide and mentor than an active teacher. The time involved in learning the content that would normally be presented in a one-hour lecture, will vary between students.

7. **I know I am a good classroom teacher, so why does the thought of doing Web courses make me feel dumb?**

7. Remember when you were a child learning to skate or ride a bike or, better yet, remember the first time you used e-mail or did a Web search? Learning any new skill makes us feel like beginners again and as adults we do not like to feel this way. Learning to teach online requires new computer skills as well as new theories of teaching. As described in question 5, start small so that you will be successful and gain confidence as you progress from novice to expert.

8. **I have taken a couple of online courses and know this is not a good learning style for me. How do I manage to become an effective online instructor?**

8. It takes patience and perseverance to become comfortable with a format that is new. Starting small and building in new experiences and methods into courses will help you become more comfortable and confident. Talk to colleagues who feel the same and see if you can find common concerns for your discomfort so that you can coach each other in becoming more comfortable.

9. **How much time does it take to convert classroom material to a Web-based offering?**

9. The first step in the conversion of traditional content to a Web-based format is to decide on the Web course tool that will be used (see Chapter 10). This may be an institutional decision and beyond your control. Once decided, however, the instructor must develop a plan that includes the basic structure of the course. Once the basic structure has been developed, the instructor can "build" the course using the options in the available Web course tool. The time involved in conversion of content to a Web-based format includes the conversion to HTML (Hypertext Markup Language), the time involved in uploading the converted content to the Web course, and the time involved in making the content accessible using the Web course options. The text based content can be easily converted to a Web-based format (HTML) by either choosing the "save as Web page" option of most current word processors or by using an HTML editor (e.g., Netscape Composer). On average, it should take 5 hours of development time for each course hour in order to convert traditional content to a Web-based

format (e.g., a 3 credit course = 15 hours). This time commitment will vary with the complexity of the course content (e.g., documents with mathematical and statistical symbols are much harder and more time consuming to convert to HTML), and the instructor's experience in developing online courses.

10. Can synchronous learning be used in staff development?

10. Setting up times for synchronous learning or chat rooms should include consideration of when the learners and instructor can best make this live connection. This can be a challenge when staff work varying hours and shifts. Careful up-front planning needs to take place prior to the course start date and publishing chat room time(s) well in advance is important for both staff and managers to arrange to be available. Also, make sure that chat room discussions add an important learning opportunity so that staff, managers, and instructor value the experience.

11. Do students' expectations of faculty differ for e-learning?

11. Students still expect the faculty to have expertise in the topic but also expect the instructor to have knowledge of where resources can be found. They also expect the instructor to know how to conduct online learning

12. Do faculty expectations of the student differ?

12. Overall, faculty will continue to expect students to contribute to the course dialogue, attend course meetings, and complete course assignments. Faculty who are experienced online instructors tend to expect a higher level of independent, self-directed learning from students than in a traditional format. They move from pedagogy to androgogy in their views and methods. They expect students to interact using the synchronous and asynchronous options available in the course. While class rolls no longer become relevant from a traditional perspective (except in a synchronous meeting such as online chat), faculty can, and will, electronically track student access to the course and the level of activity.

13. What new technical skills do online faculty need?

13. Faculty must develop a working knowledge of basic computer skills to include managing files and directories as well as the application of word processing, database, and spreadsheet software. In addition, other desirable skills include downloading and uploading files, using file compression software (e.g., WinZip, PKZip, Stuffit), creating Web-ready material using an HTML editor, converting computer-based slide presentations (e.g., PowerPoint) to a Web-based format, developing a working knowledge of at least one Web course tool (e.g., WebCT,

Blackboard). Faculty may also need to master the protocol for accessing the Internet from home or while traveling in order to participate in the course(s) anywhere/anytime.

14. How does course planning and development differ for online courses?

14. Planning for an online course requires that the instructor not only develop the content and the strategies for delivery of the content, but also the structure of the Web course itself. Each course tool (e.g., WebCT, Blackboard) has its unique approach to organizing the content into a manageable structure for easy access by the student. The instructor must develop a schematic of the Web course (either imagined or on paper), prior to creating the structure online. Once developed, the structure can then act as a template for subsequent online courses. Some institutions may mandate a specific online course structure while others may allow the instructor the freedom to personalize the structure of the online course.

15. How important is time management for the instructor moving to an e-learning environment?

15. Time management is critical. Online courses can require a high degree of maintenance especially when students are required to engage in threaded discussions and electronic submission of assignments. Online instructors should employ a time management system that enhances their ability to "keep up" with the message traffic and grading of assignments, along with all their other obligations. It is very easy to become overwhelmed with student interaction in an online course, especially if the content promotes lively discussion and an expectation by the student of a timely response by the instructor.

16. Will my philosophy of teaching and learning have to change to become a successful e-learning instructor?

16. The traditional classroom setting generally involves a pedagogical approach to teaching and learning with the instructor actively managing the teaching/learning process (e.g., a lecture with students taking notes and asking questions). The online environment requires students to become much more responsible for their own learning. This change in student involvement in learning requires the instructor to employ a teaching philosophy that is more androgogy than pedagogy. In an online course, instructors become more guide and mentor once learners are oriented to the course goals, objectives, and assignments. Instructors give students the basic tools they need to learn the required content and then reinforce the learner's success through synchronous and asynchronous interaction.

RESOURCES

Golas, K. (2000). *Guidelines for designing on-line learning.* **www.aero.swri.org/tsd/publications/pdf/ 2000ITSEC_ON-LINELEARNING.pdf**

Hazari, S. I. (1998). *Evaluation and selection of Web course management tools.* **http://sunil.umd.edu/Webct**

Horton, S. (2000). *Web teaching guide: A practical approach to creating course Websites.* New Haven, CT: Yale University Press.

Landon, B. (2001). *Online educational delivery applications: A Web tool for comparative analysis.* **http://www.ctt.bc.ca/landon-line/**

Moore, G. S., Winograd, K., & Lange, D. (2001). *You can teach online: Building a creative learning environment.* New York: McGraw-Hill Higher Education.

Schweizer, H. (1999). *Designing and teaching an on-line course: Spinning your Web classroom.* Boston, MA: Allyn and Bacon.

Chapter 13: Educator Development: Curriculum and Support Considerations

1. I want to teach an online course. How do I learn how to do it?

1. Learning how to teach online is not something that comes easily to everyone. To become an online educator, you have to change your way of thinking and learning. You become a "facilitator of learning" instead of a classroom teacher. This transition often takes time and effort. You will need to educate yourself in this area to become a good online educator—do not take it for granted that because you teach well in the classroom you will be able to make the transition to online learning. If you work in a college or university, find out what the college or university offers in the line of faculty development. Look for courses online to teach you how to teach online. If you have never taken an online course, do so! Become familiar with a variety of learning platforms for online learning. Be flexible.

A variety of programs are available to teach you to teach online. Some are listed in Table 1.

Table 1: **Online Classes to Teach Faculty How to Teach Online**

University of Massachusetts Lowell On-line Teaching Institute http://cybered.uml.edu/cy_institutes.htm
ETeaching Institute http://eteaching.ecollege.com/index.learn?action=Online
Indiana University School of Nursing Lifelong Learning http://www.nursing.iupui.edu/LifelongLearning/default.asp
ECollege http://www.ecollege.com/
Get Educated: Guide to programs that teach instructors how to teach online http://www.geteducated.com/articles/teach2000.htm

2. Why do we have to teach online courses? Why can't we just keep doing what we are doing?

2. Change is difficult! We can all attest to that. There are many reasons why we are feeling the pressure to teach online. With the fast pace of technology, and a variety of educational tools available online, it is the "in" thing to do. The question here is that if you believe you "have to teach online courses" you probably are not ready to do it. No one should be forced to teach online if they feel uncomfortable.

Students who are recent graduates from high school or college expect different teaching strategies than educators who have been teaching for several years in a lecture format. Students get restless and leave classes when they are bored with classroom lectures. This may be due to the fact that many of them have been raised on computers with graphics, animation, and visuals as entertainment. For these learners, asking them to sit, listen, and be still is asking them to do something that may not be their best way of learning. However, classroom lecture is our most comfortable way of teaching. So how do we change to meet the new generation of students' learning needs?

If we do not teach the way the students want to be taught, we are at risk of losing valuable assets in both colleges and healthcare institutions. Not only may our student numbers decline, but also we will lose the reputation of teaching using the "latest" strategies. In the competition for learners, revenue is dependent on reaching a market that can provide financial opportunities.

3. *I've heard teaching an online course is time consuming and you don't get paid any more for it. What's in it for me?*

3. Yes, the preparation for an online course takes many hours. Rewards and compensation in online teaching differ at every institution. This is something you may want to find out before you invest time and energy in an online course. Do you get any release time or compensation if you develop an online course? Do you get a "development fee" for the first time you teach a class? Are you paid based on enrollment in the class? What are the practices and guidelines related to promotion, tenure, merit, or career advancement?

The faculty I have talked to who teach online say they do it because they love it. It is fun and exciting to have so many options available online to introduce to students. I think it is an attitude. What do you believe is in it for you? Are you doing it just because you have to or because you think it is a great way for students to learn?

4. *How long does it take to develop an online course?*

4. There are many things involved that can influence the answer to this question. How much do you know about computer technology? How much do you know about the educational platform you will be teaching in? How much do you know about searches online (if you use these in the course)? How much do you know about changing a traditional lecture course to a Web-based course? How much do you know about the start-up of a course and what you can do to stay clear of things that can sabotage the course, requiring more time and energy? If you have never taught an online course, it will take you anywhere from 6 months to a year to adequately prepare yourself to teach a course and to develop a course online. Depending on how you want to develop the course also depends on how much time you want to spend on it. Interactive activities should always be included and these may take time to consider.

5. What type of courses can go online?

5. This depends on the course objectives. Almost any course can go online, except clinical experiences. What outcomes do you want to achieve and how will Web-based learning help you achieve them? Some faculty believe it is easier to have online courses that are composed of basic knowledge so they can test recall of information, knowledge of dates, events, places, knowledge of major ideas, mastery of subject matter by listing, defining, describing, or labeling. However, more advanced courses that test comprehension, application, and analysis can be developed with a variety of interactive strategies available on the Internet. If you are creative in classroom instruction, this creativity will be seen in online courses you develop as well.

6. Who decides which courses go online and how is this decision made?

6. This very complex question will be answered from two perspectives: cognitive decision or theoretical approach. The delivery method of a course is considered a teaching strategy. So, in view of this approach, any faculty should be able to decide to teach a course online. However, this is not always the case.

Colleges or healthcare agencies may give educators the choice on how to teach a course. It may be considered "academic freedom" for the educator to decide how to "teach" a class.

Some colleges have another decision-making process in place. A curriculum committee may choose which classes may go online based on the needs of the faculty and students. A committee for online learning may be in place that determines and monitors courses online.

Administrative input must also be considered. This could relate to cost, student needs, vision of the university, college, or healthcare agency, and availability of technical support. Administration may decide which courses to teach online based on budgetary constraints, scheduling needs, and faculty workloads.

Which class can go online "theoretically" is a different question. This depends on the objectives of the course and how the faculty wants to teach a course. Essentially, any course could be taught online, if you wish to develop the course. Courses that cannot go online are usually those that involve clinical experience, such as clinical rotations in nursing and other allied health fields.

7. How is online learning interactive?

7. Interactive is defined as acting upon each other. Interactive learning gets students involved in activities that enhance learning rather than passively listening to a lecture. This activity can be reading, writing, discussing, solving a problem, or responding to questions that require more than factual answers. The idea is to get students thinking about the material. The act of learning is never passive. As faculty, when we prepare to "teach," we learn actively by preparing lecture notes, reading, comparing what we have read with our experiences, synthesizing the information into coherent notes, and developing examples that illustrate the concept. We then use this understanding to lecture to students depriving them of their own journey of discovery. By carefully involving the students in learning, we can increase student depth of understanding of the material, increase student comfort with the material, and improve student confidence. Many disciplines value active learning through laboratories or programming projects.

In online learning, faculty must include interactive activities to facilitate learning rather than focus on what to teach. This can be achieved through a variety of activities like forum discussions, bulletin board postings, e-mail communications, and listservs. Teaching strategies to promote interactive learning can include activities like Web cast, role playing, case studies, online debates, drill and practice, scavenger hunts, guided research activities, learning games, brainstorming, and a variety of other activities that encourage creativity in learning and sharing of ideas.

8. If I teach an online course, what kind of technology support should I expect?

8. Technology support varies. This is something you should address when you first consider doing an online course. The development of a good online course requires a team of "experts" who are committed to the development of a quality course. The instruction team members may include the educator, instructional designer, librarian, learning resources coordinator, multimedia developer, Webmaster, video producer, copyright specialist, bookstore manager, student mentors, teaching assistants, graphics designers, and programmer, to name a few. Each of these people plays a key role in the development of the online course.

Another part of "technology support" is faculty development. It is important to ask what the institution will support in your own development of knowledge in online education. If you take classes to learn how to teach online, who will pay for them? Will you get release time to go to these classes to learn how to teach online?

9. Do I have to be a computer "guru" to teach an online course?

9. No, you do not have to be a guru in computers—however, you have to be willing to learn about the methodology of online teaching. You must be open to learning new things and staying abreast of new knowledge related to online education. Your computer knowledge will increase as you work with the technology and eventually you may be known as the "guru" of online learning. This happens very subtly and will surprise you! With experience, you will eventually know more than you ever thought possible.

10. Before I commit to teaching an online course, what should I know?

10. You must know the platform that your institution supports—if they support more than one—and the impact that this will have on support. You should know basic word processing. And you should know how to access information on the Internet, a valuable source to enhance learning. Above all, you should be able to practice good communication skills through the online medium with special attention to "netiquette."

11. Is there an "art" to online teaching?

11. There is definitely an "art" to online teaching. The art of online teaching comes from questions like "what do we know about online teaching?" What is your personal knowledge about online teaching? How do you acquire knowledge? And what about ethical considerations in online learning that we need to address? Caring for students is another issue of the "art" of online teaching. The student should be the priority—are we giving students the best possible online course based on our scholarship as educators?

Online teaching requires a transition from being a teacher to being a facilitator of learning. Quality education must be at the forefront of all online courses. It is having the skill to be able to communicate with students without touching or seeing them. It requires an art to care for the student through minimal sensory connection. It is knowing how to troubleshoot and prevent problems before they happen. The art of online learning is being proactive and supportive of students even more than in the traditional classroom setting. It is imperative to build a trusting relationship with students who you may never "put your eyes on." These things may be difficult to do and not all faculty are capable of transcending these obstacles.

12. How do I learn all the technological aspects of the learning platform? Who teaches me?

12. In many instances, you will have to be proactive and teach yourself. You will have to find ways to learn based on your own learning needs. The learning management systems for online learning (see Section 3) usually have a tutorial to assist faculty in the development of online courses. However, hands on experience with a one on one instructor is very helpful. This support varies by institution. If you are lucky enough to have a progressive institution with technological support for educators, you may have classes available to you for the asking. Check with your education department or faculty development resources office. In the event these are not available, do a search on the Internet for help available. You may be able to find online classes to assist you in online learning and the platform you use.

13. What are some key points I should know when teaching an online course?

13.
- Communicate with students!
- Be organized.
- Plan ahead.
- Expect technological failures in the system.
- Do not expect everything to be perfect— plan on glitches.
- Be flexible.
- Do not react—be proactive!

14. What are the usual complaints that students have in online courses?

14. Students often have problems with the initial stages of online learning such as how to log on, upgrading their computers, or fear of the unknown. Many may feel isolated and feel they do not have anyone to work with or help them. This can be very easily alleviated with careful planning and communication. Another problem identified with students is procrastination.

15. How can I become certified in online teaching and learning?

15. A certification program is a program of study that provides learners with a set of specific competencies. It usually involves several courses but is less than a "degree" program. It may be an intensive program or divided over time in several courses. Certificate programs are usually completed within 3–9 months. There are several courses available to become certified in online learning. When choosing a program, review the program objectives, competencies, and learning outcomes. Determine if residency is required. Analyze who is teaching the program—is there an advisory board that maintains quality? Determine if contact hours for continuing education are awarded. The certificate is not a license but is recognition of your accomplishments.

16. What resources are available to me to help me learn how to teach online?

16. A variety of Web pages online can assist you in planning, developing, implementing, and evaluating online learning. Books are available to help with online learning/teaching also. The resource section of this chapter offers several books that are helpful to nurse educators.

17. If I develop this course, to whom does it belong?

17. Questions related to "intellectual property" are very important to ask. The new capabilities offered by distance learning environments have created controversy regarding ownership of online materials. The development of policies for ownership of online courses has been a major issue for many colleges and universities. Some institutions retain ownership themselves; some allow faculty members to retain ownership; and some rely on arrangements under which ownership is shared. (See Chapter 34 for further information).

Recently, Stevens Institute of Technology faculty members approved an intellectual property policy for online education. The policy gives many of the rights and rewards for courses to the faculty members who develop them. Under the policy, faculty members at the New Jersey institution are paid to develop online courses, will own the material in the courses they develop, and will control how and when that material can be used. The institution will control the copyrights of the online courses and will manage the courses' distribution. In return for giving up the copyright on a course, a faculty member will receive a third of the revenue whenever a business or other institution purchases use of the course (**http://chronicle.merit.edu/free/2000/11/2000112201u.htm**).

18. How do I work with colleagues who resist teaching online?

18. Resistance to online teaching is seen across campuses and in healthcare agencies for a variety of reasons including:

- "faceless" teaching,

- fear of the imminent replacement of faculty by computers,

- diffusion of value traditionally placed on getting a degree,

- faculty culture,

- lack of an adequate time-frame to implement online courses,

- distance learners who lack independent learning skills and local library resources,

- lack of formalized agreements to sustain program commitment through difficulties and problems,

- high cost of materials,

- increased time required for both online contacts and preparation of materials/activities,

- failure of technology and the learning system,

- non-educational considerations take precedence over educational priorities,

- resistance to change, and

- lack of technological assistance.

We are embarking on a new frontier in online education. Many of us have no one with whom to share successes or failure. Sometimes, we feel like we are isolated and alone in developing this process. Change is a difficult thing to initiate and if you are the first to develop an online course, you will have to consider all the change theories you have ever learned and implement them in this process.

Lewin's Change Theory is one that may be used to implement a plan for "resistance to online teaching." Faculty or instructors need to be aware of the need for online learning; discuss the pros and cons. The issue is identified and discussed. Everyone can be heard and their voices respected. Disequilibrium is introduced to the organization. A need for change is identified. Faculty collect information on online learning. This can be done individually or through committee work. Administration will have a direct impact on this process. All the pros and cons of online learning should be considered. A specific proactive objective should be the focus. A decision is made and a plan implemented. This decision can be:

1) Who teaches online courses?

2) Who decides which classes can go online?

3) What about faculty workload?

4) What about philosophical viewpoints that oppose online learning?

5) What about intellectual property?

6) What about compensation or release time?

Once the topics of concern are discussed and decisions are made, the group should move forward in implementing the decisions. Restraining forces (those against the decision) will continue to influence the driving forces (those who support the decision). Change is established once equilibrium is restored.

As a leader in this process, keep in mind Covey's (1990) *7 Habits* as he relates them to personal change:

1. Remain proactive—Do not react. Present information logically and with justification of the discussion.

2. Begin with the end in mind—Where do you want to see online education going in the program/ curriculum?

3. Put first things first—What is the most important thing you need to take care of now? What will influence the school or program? What needs to be discussed or is just being rehashed over and over again? What system is already in place that can answer some of the questions?

4. Think win/win—Come up with solutions that can benefit everyone. If faculty are concerned that online courses are competitive with traditional courses, put a cap on the online course. Team-teach to include faculty who are not teaching online.

5. Seek first to understand, then to be understood— Consider the fears that your cohorts are experiencing. If they have not taken the time to educate themselves, their fears are usually unfounded. Work with them— try to understand their concerns.

6. Synergize—Come up with new solutions and creative

answers to the issues. There are no black and white answers. Work together.

7. Sharpen the saw—Go back, re-think, take care of you. Consider the environment you are working in. Maybe you have outgrown the facility and it is time to go somewhere that you can "spread your wings and fly."

RESOURCES

Covey, S. (1990). *The 7 habits of highly effective people: Powerful lessons in personal change.* New York: Simon & Schuster.

Moore, G., Winograd, K., & Lange, D. (2001). *You can teach online: The McGraw Hill guide to building a creative learning environment.* New York: McGraw Hill.

Palloff, R., & Pratt, K. (2001). *Lessons from the cyberspace classroom: The realities of online teaching.* San Francisco: Jossey-Bass.

Hanna, D., Glowacki-Dudka, M., & Conceicao-Runlee, S. (2000). *147 practical tips for teaching online groups: Essentials of Web-based education.* Madison, WI: Atwood Publishing.

Schor Ko, S., & Rossen, S. (2000). *Teaching online: A practical guide.* Boston: Houghton Mifflin Co.

Horton, W. (2000). *Designing Web-based training: How to teach anyone, anything, anywhere, anytime.* New York: John Wiley & Sons.

Chapter 14: *How Will My Role Change When I Teach on the Web?*

1. Will my role as educator change when I teach on the Web?

1. Yes, you will find that your role as an educator will change when you teach on the Web. You will have limited, or maybe no, face-to-face contact with the students that you are teaching. Most interaction with students will occur electronically and asynchronously. You will be less likely to be the primary source of information for the students in a course.

2. As an educator teaching a Web course, what becomes my primary role with students?

2. Instead of being a primary source of information for students, you become a facilitator of student learning. You will identify expected outcomes for student learning and design learning experiences that will encourage students to become actively involved in the learning process, meet their learning goals, and achieve the expected outcomes. Providing frequent feedback to students is an essential part of this role.

3. What does it mean to "facilitate" student learning?

3. Facilitating student learning means that you guide students as they assume responsibility for identifying their own learning needs and become self-directed in the process they use to achieve the expected outcomes of the course.

4. What teaching behaviors do I need to adopt as a facilitator of student learning?

4. You will need to clearly identify expected outcomes and learning activities so that students will know what is expected of them in the course. Since most Web teaching will occur asynchronously, you will also need to be able to manage online discussion and effectively communicate with students with minimal face-to-face interaction. The timeliness of communication with students is important to the success of Web teaching. Establishing and communicating evaluation criteria and providing prompt student feedback on performance are other essential teaching behaviors.

5. I am used to lecturing in the classroom. How can I transfer this teaching style to the Web?

5. First of all, no matter how tempting it may be, do *not* place your lectures word-for-word on the Web. This does not promote active student learning. Instead, use the content of your lectures to identify "chunks" of content and design learning modules that will help students explore the concepts related to the content. For example, learning modules may contain learning objectives, reading assignments (texts, journals, and online resources), study questions, and examples of learning activities that students can complete to help them apply the content.

6. **What can I do to assure myself that students are learning what they need in a Web course?**

6. When teaching a Web course, it is important to assess student learning throughout the course. To help you evaluate student learning build in periodic formative evaluation techniques. For example, you can evaluate student learning through online discussion, short quizzes, writing assignments, and case study assignments that require application of the content.

7. **How do I develop a teaching/learning relationship with students if I do not regularly meet with them in the classroom?**

7. You will build these relationships through other means—primarily through the use of online discussion, e-mail, and the telephone. Prompt responses to student inquiries will help foster positive student/faculty interactions. Establishing regular electronic and telephone "office" hours will help students know when you can be easily contacted.

8. **How do I actively involve students in the learning process in a Web course?**

8. While textbooks, journals, and Web-based resources can be important sources of information, avoid relying solely on reading assignments to promote student learning in a Web course. To get students actively involved in the learning process, design learning activities that require them to apply the content they are studying. Group learning activities, debates, case studies, and critical thinking exercises are examples of learning activities that require interaction and promote active involvement in the learning process.

9. **How can I identify "at-risk" students in a Web course early enough to intervene?**

9. Students who are "at-risk" in a Web course are likely to be those who lack the necessary discipline for self-directed learning or those who are overwhelmed with the technology. These factors will begin to emerge in the first two to three weeks of the course. Require students to interact with you and each other during the first couple of weeks in the course so that you can assess their level of course involvement. Individually contact students whose participation is not at an acceptable level to further assess the problem.

10. **What methods can I use to communicate with students?**

10. You can interact with students through asynchronous communication such as online discussion, listserv, and individual e-mail. Synchronous communication can be achieved through the use of chat rooms and, of course, the telephone.

11. What is my role in facilitating asynchronous online discussion?

11. Your role is primarily one of establishing the purpose for the online discussion and ensuring that students initiate and participate in the discussion. As the discussion develops online, you may occasionally find it necessary to refocus discussion, summarize key concepts, and correct any factual errors that students may post about the topic under discussion. You will also want to encourage students in the course who are reluctant to participate in the discussion.

12. Do I need to respond to every comment students post for online discussion?

12. No, it is not necessary or even desirable to respond to every comment that students post. The students will respond to each other's comments and you can comment when necessary to help guide the discussion. You do not want to dominate the online discussion.

13. What time management concerns will I need to consider when I begin teaching a Web course?

13. When teaching a Web course, you can easily find yourself responding to student e-mail, phone calls, and Web postings seven days a week! This is certainly not necessary, but it is easy to fall into this pattern if you do not organize your time prior to teaching the course. Common time management concerns include managing online communication with students and providing student feedback in a timely manner.

14. How can I manage the volume of e-mail I will receive from students?

14. Before the course begins, decide when and how often you are going to respond to student e-mail and communicate this to students so they know when to anticipate a reply. Some faculty choose to organize student e-mail by establishing an e-mail account for the course so that student e-mail is automatically sorted from other work or personal e-mail messages. I also establish individual file folders for each student, so that I can save all pertinent e-mail messages and assignments received from the student during the course.

15. How can I manage my time most effectively?

15. Prior to teaching the course think through when you will be available for electronic office hours, when you will respond to student e-mail, and when you will review and respond to any online discussion postings. Consider developing standardized replies to the most commonly asked questions that you can save in an electronic file and individualize for quick responses to student questions. Use distribution lists or group e-mail to respond to students whenever appropriate. Blocking out intervals of time each week to attend to the course can help keep you organized from week to week while teaching the course.

16. Will e-learning make positions for educators obsolete?

16. No. Quality e-learning requires educators who are experts at designing learning experiences to achieve specific, desired outcomes. E-learning actually demands more faculty time than classroom teaching because of the amount of individualized student/faculty interaction. While e-learning will not make positions for educators obsolete, it will reshape the role of the educator and the learning environment.

17. How much time will I spend teaching online vs. teaching in the classroom?

17. You can anticipate spending more time teaching a course online than you would spend teaching it in the classroom. The amount of time you spend teaching an online course can actually double, but will vary depending upon the course content, level of student, and number of students. This extra time demand is primarily because of the increased interaction that you will experience with the students in the course.

18. What is the ideal class size for Web courses?

18. Ideal class size will vary depending upon the nature of the course and level of student. A class size of 20–25 students is usually manageable. With larger numbers of students, faculty can quickly become overwhelmed with the amount of e-mail and student interaction that the increased numbers will generate.

19. Will administrators expect me to teach more students?

19. Administrators may expect you to teach more students in Web courses; these are usually administrators who do not have firsthand experience teaching a Web course. It is becoming evident that the primary attraction to e-learning is the flexibility and access that it affords students, with the potential for increasing student enrollment in the institution. When large numbers of students are placed in course sections, the quality of the educational experience deteriorates, leading to faculty and student dissatisfaction. Most accrediting bodies within higher education have established criteria for quality e-learning experiences with which administrators and faculty need to be familiar.

20. How will I balance my other educator roles if I am teaching on the Web?

20. It is possible to balance the roles of teaching, research, and service when you teach on the Web. The schedule flexibility that you have when teaching Web courses can help you manage your time to incorporate research and service activities. The important thing is to carefully plan and organize Web teaching responsibilities to incorporate these activities. For example, if you wish to use time on Thursdays to pursue scholarship and

Wednesday mornings to provide community service, you can schedule Web teaching activities for other times during the week. Remember, when you are teaching on the Web, you can keep in touch with students from anywhere in the world, even while you are attending professional conferences.

RESOURCES

Halstead, J. A., & Coudret, N. (2000). Implementing Web-based instruction in a school of nursing: Implications for faculty and students. *Journal of Professional Nursing*, 16(5), 273–281.

Moore, G., Winograd, K., & Lange, D. (2001). *You can teach on-line: The McGraw Hill guide to building a creative learning environment.* Amherst, MA: McGraw Hill.

Section 5:
E-Learners

E-learning is a new world for learners, too. Learners in the digital age learn in new ways, are balancing multiple responsibilities, have diverse backgrounds, and are seeking career development and advancement. They require access to education at convenient times, and just-in-time. On their way to becoming e-learners, learners will need orientation to basic technology, the course tools, and their role as e-learners. They also need access to a host of online academic and non-academic services such as registration, advising, career planning and tutoring, scholarships, and course materials. The authors of the chapters in this unit explain how to assess learners' needs, the importance of understanding learners' expectations, how to plan for orientation, and the types of required learner support services.

15. **Identifying Learner Needs and Expectations**
Carol McDougall, MSN, RN
Richard Hernandez, DrPH, RRT

16. **Learner Support**
Carla Mueller PhD, RN

17. **Orienting E-Learners to Technology and New Roles**
Carla Mueller PhD, RN

Chapter 15: *Identifying Learner Needs and Expectations*

1. What is learner assessment?

1. Learner assessment for Web-based courses not only includes finding out what the learner needs to know, but also identifying what is the learner's comfort and ability to be successful in online learning. Since online learning requires the student to be an active participant in the learning experience, the instructor must know the learner's ability to be successful.

2. What should I assess about learners?

2. E-learning differs from the traditional classroom setting. Instructors need to know something about the learner's ability to learn in a non-classroom setting. It is also helpful to know the learner's ability to be self-directed. Of course, the instructor also needs to know the learner's comfort with using a computer, and the Web, and with the dynamics of online learning.

3. Why is leaner assessment important?

3. E-learning is a new method of learning for most students, and as instructors we want students to be successful. Having students complete a learning assessment prior to beginning an online program helps us to identify opportunities to assist them. The student also has the opportunity to identify his/her own strengths and weaknesses and therefore seek needed resources. In some cases, learning assessment may identify learners who are at very high risk for failure in online learning and these students will need additional onsite support from faculty.

4. How does identifying learner needs differ for e-learning?

4. Traditional methods of identifying learning needs use paper surveys/questionnaires and focus groups. While these methods can be used for e-learning, completing online learning assessments gives the instructors and learners more insight into their needs to be successful online learners. Since this is such a new method of learning for most students, personal knowledge of learning style and personal need for classroom-student-teacher interaction also is important.

5. Are there learner assessment tools already developed that I can use?

5. The Internet has many learner assessment tools that assess learners' abilities in a variety of areas. Some good ones address personality profiles (**www.Keirsey.com**) while others address learning styles, computer skills, and almost anything else you want to assess (e.g., **www.Emode.com**; **www.On-linelearning.com**; **www.learningcircuits.org**). I have found ones that are

listed on university Web sites are the most reliable. Since Web addresses change, I suggest using a search engine such as Google.com and entering such phrases as "online learning style assessment tools."

6. *How do I convert learner needs surveys to an online environment in a traditional hospital-based inservice setting?*

6. It is important to know what network technical system support you have in the setting. Will surveys be able to be completed on line and returned or do they need to be printed and mailed back? Will online completed surveys be summarized for you? Surveys online need to be concise so it is important to make sure the question obtains the information you want. Again, there are some excellent resources on survey development that can be found on the Web.

7. *Are there surveys or assessment tools that help identify the learners' computer skills?*

7. There are many assessment surveys that can be found online to assess computer skills. Most can be downloaded and printed for the novice. Some are geared to educational levels, which is very helpful for staff development educators who have a wide variation in educational backgrounds to consider. Using a search engine such as Google and entering "online learning style assessment tools" or "learning style questionnaires" will bring up a variety of tools.

8. *How do educators address the diversity of learner computer skills?*

8. This can be a challenge if the group's skills are very diverse. One very helpful method is to have all the learners come together for an onsite introduction to the course. If possible, have classroom meetings for those who need additional assistance. Having learners complete computer skills surveys prior to starting the course can help the instructor build additional online assistance into the course for those who need it. On the other hand, be prepared to add other learning opportunities for proficient online learners so that they remain engaged and challenged.

9. *How do I help the "technically challenged" individual become comfortable with e-learning?*

9. Having an onsite introduction to the course can help the "technically challenged" student become familiar with online learning. Offering basic computer skills training is also helpful. In staff development this is particularly a problem with some categories of learners. When we first introduced computer-based learning in the hospital, we teamed persons who were comfortable with those who weren't. They learned from each other as well as felt supported when the educators could not be present.

10. *Are expectations of students different in online learning as opposed to classroom learning?*

10. The fundamental difference between online learning and the traditional classroom format is the loss of face-to-face interaction. Students in a traditional classroom setting expect immediate feedback from instructors, and many times react to both verbal and non-verbal cues. Student expectations in an online environment will differ depending on the type of synchronous and asynchronous interaction used. Since students can no longer depend on the non-verbal cues of the instructor (body language), they expect the online interaction to be clear, concise, and as free of ambiguity as possible. Students' expectations of the faculty availability can increase when compared to a classroom setting since students can post questions and comments on a 24 hour a day, 7 day a week basis instead of only during a defined classroom period.

11. *Employees within hospital settings are not accustomed to anytime/anywhere learning. What strategies can staff development educators use to encourage this method of learning?*

11. Starting with something that is fun, innovative, and short is a good way! The value of the offering is also very important. If staff believe that the information enhances their working knowledge they may be more willing to use online learning opportunities. When staff see that they can do online learning at their choice of time and not have to give up valued days off, their approach to this method of learning changes. Staff development educators as well as managers need to acknowledge that this is a new method of learning and recognize staff who take a leadership role.

12. *In staff development, learners are used to work-related programs being offered during work hours. How does the learner change to using his/her own time or combination of paid and own time?*

12. This has been a challenge for us. Our first venture into online learning used a commercial product that the hospital bought for the annual regulatory review requirements. While staff loved the format, they resisted doing it on their own time since they needed to be in the hospital to access the program. As we have progressed with newer programming, we now have access to these programs over the hospital Intranet. Staff can now access the Intranet off site. Each manager assigns staff a date to complete these programs (usually at the annual performance review) so staff use a combination of paid time and their personal time, having been given the accountability to complete the program prior to the review date. Purchasing online continuing education and providing staff free time to do it is seen as a "perk" by many staff and makes staff feel appreciated and supported.

13. *How much time do learners need to complete e-learning courses?*

13. E-learning courses vary in length depending on the amount and type of synchronous and asynchronous activities along with the level of interactivity. Courses that only involve the reading of text-based material will take less time to complete than courses with a high level of interactivity. A text-based course could be completed at the student's convenience and in a short time frame. Courses could also be developed that include activities spread out over a traditional semester as well. One rule of thumb would be that the greater the level of interaction and instructor management, the longer it would take to complete an online course.

14. *Can a learner who needs a teacher-directed environment be successful in e-learning?*

14. Online courses tend to be developed using a self-directed learning model that minimizes student/teacher interaction. However, online courses can also include a high degree of student/teacher interaction. One of the advantages of a well-developed online course is the potential for improved communication between students and teachers through synchronous and asynchronous interaction. Using online threaded discussions, for example, students have access to instructors (and other students) virtually 24 hours a day, 7 days a week. Online chat rooms can be used to hold planned, and impromptu, class sessions. In order to accommodate the student who works best in a teacher-directed environment, the online course would need to include options for promoting communication and interaction.

15. *What effect does the e-learning environment have on expectations of learner responsibility and interactivity?*

15. It is not uncommon for instructors to rely heavily on asynchronous discussion groups to generate ongoing interaction between the instructor and students as well as between students. Online courses require a greater investment in self-directed learning by the student than most traditional classroom settings, and thus, a greater burden is placed on the student to seek out learning opportunities. The instructor acts more as a guide for students and less as an all-knowing "sage." There is an ongoing debate as to whether student contributions to an electronic discussion group should be mandatory or voluntary. Those who advocate mandatory posting to an electronic discussion group argue that it is the only way to ensure that students ask questions and submit comments on a consistent basis. Those who advocate a voluntary approach argue that students should feel free to interact at their leisure, and when they do, their communication will be of a higher quality. The decision to mandate or allow voluntary online interaction should be a decision made by the instructor taking into consideration the course content, the importance of interaction to the course goals and objectives, and the type of students enrolled in the course.

16. How does one develop a user-friendly e-learning environment for the learner?

16. The key to a user-friendly e-learning environment is the choice of Web course tools and the instructor's mastery of those tools. The instructor may or may not be the course designer, but once the course is made available to the students, the instructor then becomes responsible for ensuring that students feel comfortable using the course environment, and that learning is maximized. This requires the instructor to master the basic course management knowledge and skills. This can be accomplished through a comprehensive faculty development program that prepares faculty to be effective instructors within the e-learning environment.

17. What are some strategies for maximizing retention in e-learning courses?

17. Online courses can be developed to maximize student retention. The course syllabus should be constructed using a clear and concise format that clearly delineates the instructor's expectations, course requirements, and deadlines. Assignments can be constructed to include text, slides (e.g., PowerPoint) and can be linked to supplemental material on the Web. Assignments can also be preceded or followed by synchronous (e.g., online chat) or asynchronous (e.g., threaded discussion) interaction that can reinforce study material. Online exams can be constructed so that students get feedback concerning their answers and explanations as to why one answer is more correct than another. Mechanisms can be available for students to access instructors by phone as a means of supplementing online interaction.

RESOURCES

Golas, K. (2000). *Guidelines for designing on-line learning.* **www.aero.swri.org/tsd/publications/pdf/ 2000ITSEC_ON-LINELEARNING.pdf**

Hazari, S. I. (1998). *Evaluation and selection of Web course management tools.* **http://sunil.umd.edu/Webct**

Horton, S. (2000). *Web teaching guide: A practical approach to creating course Websites.* New Haven, CT: Yale University Press.

Landon, B. (2001). *Online educational delivery applications: A Web tool for comparative analysis.* **http://www.ctt.bc.ca/landon-line/**

Moore, G. S., Winograd, K., & Lange, D. (2001). *You can teach online: Building a creative learning environment.* New York: McGraw-Hill Higher Education.

Schweizer, H. (1999). *Designing and teaching an online course: Spinning your Web classroom.* Boston, MA: Allyn and Bacon.

Chapter 16: *Learner Support*

1. How do I prepare students to be successful e-learners?

2. What "academic" support systems will learners need in an online course?

3. What "non-academic" support systems will students taking an online course need?

4. Should learner support be centralized or localized?

1. Introduction of students to expectations of e-learning is critical to learner success. Students need to be aware of computer requirements, computer-related skills, course deadlines, and the amount of work required for the course. Students sometimes have the misconception that e-learning is "independent study" and does not have firm deadlines. While some courses are structured as independent study courses, many e-learning courses have deadlines for assignments. In order to foster interaction and collaboration, students need to be working with the material at the same time. This collaboration enhances learning, but is often a surprise to some students new to e-learning who expect to be working on their own. Discuss with students the skills needed to be successful such as resourcefulness, coping skills, strong writing skills, ability to work independently, time management and organizational skills, and the willingness to take responsibility for their own learning.

2. Traditional academic support systems will be needed for e-learners such as tutoring, library access, assistance with study and learning skills, and strategies to enhance academic self-concept. These should be offered via telephone, e-mail, discussion board, or chat room. Support services need to be offered outside the traditional 8:30 a.m.–5:00 p.m. time frame since e-learners may be working during the day or be located in different time zones.

3. Non-academic support systems needed include advising (course selection), vocational guidance, administrative support (registration, financial aid, career advising, bookstore), and problem solving (institution-related, study, time, personal problems). As noted previously, these support services need to be offered in a variety of delivery modes and outside the traditional timeframe since e-learners may be working during the day or be located in different time zones.

4. Learner support can be offered in either manner, but support is more efficient when it is centralized. Students can contact a single location for assistance and not have to search multiple sources of information or contact multiple individuals for assistance. Multiple contacts serve as a source of frustration for students as they begin to worry that no one will be able to help them. Faculty members should serve as an initial resource to provide student support for common, easily solved problems. However, faculty should not be responsible for complex, difficult problems since their primary focus is teaching, not technology.

5. What are the best ways to provide learner support?

5. Learner support is best provided via multiple avenues. A distance learning student manual can serve as a handy reference and be provided in print or online prior to the beginning of classes. Frequently asked questions (FAQs) and their solutions can be posted on a Web page. Response to questions via e-mail or fax back service can also be useful. However, nothing replaces talking to a "real person" when students are frustrated and having difficulty. The ability to talk to a person either via the telephone or chat room in real-time is crucial to learner support.

6. What learner supports should be built into delivery of the program?

6. Traditional learner supports should be built into the program such as academic advising, tutoring, and career services; as well as those needed specifically for distance learners such as increased assistance with computer-related problems and distance learning courseware.

7. How long does it take to develop these support systems?

7. Several months should be allowed for development and coordination of support services. People in the support services are used to dealing with on-campus students and are often not familiar with distance learning. They will need assistance to understand the needs of distance learners and the best way to provide support to distance learners.

8. Does student support need to be available 24/7?

8. Student support ideally should be offered 24 hours a day/7 days a week, especially for computer-related support. However, this is not realistic for many smaller colleges, universities, and healthcare agencies. Alternatives to this are 24/7 student support during high usage times at the beginning of the semester, contracting with a company for student support related to computer technology, or developing a collaborative arrangement with another college or university using the same distance learning courseware to share personnel costs for evening and night technical support for distance learning courseware and computer technology.

9. Who should be involved in student support?

9. Student support is provided by a team of people with expertise to best serve the students' needs. Although student support may be centralized, faculty are often the first to receive questions and may be able to solve common problems, but should be prepared to refer

students to the appropriate department for additional help for complex problems. Depending on the college or university, computer-related support may be provided by the Distance Education Department or by Academic Computing, or the Information Technology Department at healthcare agencies.

10. How do I support e-learners?

10. Faculty can best support e-learners with frequent interaction both inside and outside of the course. Recent research about computer-mediated collaboration indicates that regular interaction with faculty enhances socialization into the profession. Faculty need to establish regular office hours either online or via telephone to decrease students' perception of isolation from faculty. Online office hours may be offered in synchronously via chat features of courseware (or other software such as NetMeeting) or asynchronously via a *Virtual Office* on the discussion board. An advantage to augmenting synchronous office hours with a *Virtual Office* on the discussion board is that all students get to see answers to questions raised. This is important since more than one student often has the same question, but may be too shy or afraid to raise it.

11. What course resource supports are necessary for e-learning?

11. Course resource supports necessary for e-learning include access to the Internet, a personal e-mail account that allows receipt of attachments, and library services. Library services should include electronic article reserves, online search capability, online ordering of materials (both in-library materials and inter-library loans), and access to full-text journal articles pertinent to the discipline.

12. What type of social spaces do students need online?

12. Social spaces in traditional, on-campus education such as student lounges or student centers are well established. In online courses, however, there are limited opportunities for social exchange with other students. Some students report a sense of isolation from peers and faculty when enrolled in online courses. Faculty must establish a sense of community within online courses to decrease this sense of isolation. To do this, faculty must first introduce students to one another at the beginning of the course. A good way to do this is via an initial Discussion Board assignment that contains an icebreaker activity. Opportunities for continued personal interaction outside required assignments should be provided such as virtual cafés and unmonitored chat rooms. Faculty may need to role model use of these areas and encourage student interaction since students are often uncomfortable in this format at first because of lack of familiarity.

13. How can students be assisted to develop personal and study support systems?

13. E-learners need assistance to develop personal and study support systems to overcome their perceived sense of isolation. Faculty can assist students in identifying their needs and provide suggestions for obtaining assistance when necessary. Personal support can include support from family members, previous students who can serve as role models and technology tutors, coworkers, and employers. Coworkers can be supportive of e-learners when they are aware that they are taking such classes. Coworkers' support can range from verbal encouragement to volunteering to change shifts when assignments and exams are scheduled.

Some students may need assistance in learning course content. The need for course tutors should be anticipated for lower level courses or courses where difficulty can be anticipated. Peer tutors who have previously completed the course successfully may be used, or professionals in the community may serve as study mentors. Peer study groups may be also developed within a course to provide support to students. Study groups can be given space to meet synchronously or asynchronously via the e-learning courseware. General study support systems (such as course tutors or writing assistance) are usually centralized in a Learning Resource Center. Faculty should refer students to the Learning Resource Center, but students should also be encouraged to contact the center independently to arrange the type of services that best meet their needs.

14. What support is needed for educationally disadvantaged students?

14. To facilitate success, educationally disadvantaged students need assistance prior to beginning a distance-learning program. Early identification of at-risk students can enable referral to writing, math, and tutorial services that bring them up to academic requirements. Some colleges and universities have developed a *Bridge to College* program that helps educationally disadvantaged students prepare for successful entry into college. These programs traditionally run during the summer prior to courses starting, but could be offered any time during the year if the college or university has admission several times a year.

Students who lack computer-related skills can be referred to tutorials for basic computer use; use and efficient searching of the Internet; and use of word processing, spreadsheet, and presentation software. This prevents students from having to learn these skills and course content at the same time.

15. What support is needed for students with disabilities?

15. The Department of Education has established Requirements for Accessible Electronic and Information Technology (E&IT) Design in order to support its obligations, under Sections 504 and 508 of the Rehabilitation Act of 1973, 29 U.S.C. 794 and 794d. Accessible electronic and information technology design calls for the development of information systems flexible enough to accommodate the needs of a broad range of computer users and telecommunications equipment, regardless of age or disability. Accessible Web and course design:

- Enables use of screen readers for visually impaired users

- Avoids use of tables or frames since these complicate the use of screen readers

- Titles frames (when used) with text to facilitate frame identification and navigation

- Provides a text format rather than a graphical format for Web pages

- Provides an alternative interpretation in text if a graphic is essential to navigating a site or provides vital information (such as a map or illustration) to provide users with visual disabilities access to the information

- Provides text alternatives to information provided via audio and video-streaming for students with visual and auditory disabilities

- Uses link text consisting of substantive, descriptive words that can be quickly reviewed by the user. Avoids nondescript words such as "this" or "here" that do not convey enough information about the nature of the link

- Provides alternative mechanisms for online forms (such as e-mail, voice/TTY phone numbers)

Information regarding accessible electronic and information technology design is more completely and specifically delineated at the Department of Education Web site: **http://www.ed.gov/offices/OCFO/contracts/clibrary/software.html**.

16. What support is needed for students who have English as a second language?

16. Students who have English as a second language (ESL) have found that distance learning is a good way to begin taking classes offered in English. These students have the opportunity to write out their responses and edit them using grammar and spell checking features of the word processor prior to posting their responses online. Ultimately, this increases their familiarity with the language. In the interim, they may need an in-depth introduction to the language with a course for students speaking English, assistance in using a word processing program, introduction to the grammar/spell checking features, and referral to a writing tutor. A writing tutor should be available for contact via telephone and e-mail to assist ESL students, especially for longer papers and projects. Rapid feedback is essential for these students so that they do not become lost and frustrated.

17. How can learner support influence continuation/retention in the course or program?

17. The decision to return to school is a difficult one. Students who find multiple obstacles in their path when first beginning classes or even during their first semester are likely to drop the class or finish it but not take further classes. Learner support is key to student success in the classroom and assists with retention.

RESOURCES

Bonk, C. J., & Cunningham, D. J. (1998). Searching for learner-centered, constructivist, and sociocultural components of collaborative educational learning tools. In C.J. Bonk & K. S. King (Eds.), *Electronic collaborators* (pp. 25–50). Mahway, NJ: Lawrence Erlbaum Associates.

Gibson, C. C. (1998). *Distance learners in higher education: Institutional responses for quality outcomes.* Madison, WI: Atwood Publishing.

Mueller, C. L. (2001). *Master's in nursing students' experience in a virtual classroom on the Internet.* Unpublished doctoral dissertation.

Novotny, J. (2000). *Distance education in nursing.* New York: Springer.

Oehlkers, R. (1998). Focus: Informal support. *Distance Education Systemwide Interactive Electronic Newsletter, 3*(9), 1–3.

Simpson, O. (2000). *Supporting students in open and distance learning.* Sterling, VA: Stylus Publishing.

Chapter 17: *Orienting E-Learners to Technology and New Roles*

1. *What orientation do e-learners need?*

1. Students new to e-learning need orientation to a variety of topics:

   - Assessment for e-learning readiness (e.g., learning style, time management skills, computer-related skills, writing skills)

   - Hardware requirements for e-learning

   - How to access the e-learning course

   - Using e-learning courseware (e.g. discussion board, chat room)

   - Course expectations

     - Faculty role

     - Student role

     - Course assignments

   - Support services available at the institution

2. *How can e-learners be oriented to technology?*

2. Orientation can be offered in person in a traditional on campus classroom (not realistic for e-learners widely separated by geography or hampered by time constraints), via a print manual, videotape, or the Internet. Although some students may desire a "hands-on approach," especially if their technology skills are weak, most students prefer to have orientation delivered in a mode that is convenient to them. Delivering orientation in the mode in which the course will be offered (electronically) gives the student the information as well as practice using the technology with which the course will be offered.

3. *Should orientation be required or optional?*

3. The philosophy of the institution dictates whether the orientation is required or optional. At the very least, orientation should be strongly encouraged since learner success is tied to the ability to hit the ground running when the course begins.

4. *What are the most common problems that learners have with the online learning technology?*

4.
   - Computer does not meet the requirements of the courseware

     - Aging computers may not meet the technical requirements of the courseware

     - Lack of Internet access

- Internet browser is not up-to-date

- Computer does not have the necessary software to read posted files (e.g., Word, PowerPoint, Adobe Acrobat Reader)

- Some courseware works better with IBM compatible PCs than Macintosh computers

• Learner cannot remember how to logon to the e-learning course

- Cannot remember URL

- Cannot remember User ID

- Cannot remember Password

• Learner lacks computer-related skills

- Using e-mail and opening attachments

- Searching the Internet

- Using word processing, spreadsheet, or presentation software

• Learner does not understand how to participate in a threaded discussion or chat room and does not understand the difference between them

5. What is the "learning curve" for students related to technology and e-learning?

5. Students new to e-learning experience a "learning curve" where their expectations of learning in the traditional classroom clash with the realities of learning online. There is also a "learning curve" for students related to use of computer technology in a new way. Learning how to use the e-learning courseware consumes a great deal of new students' time for the first two weeks of the course.

6. When does this "learning curve" begin to flatten out?

6. The "learning curve" begins go down after the first two weeks of a 15-week course and flattens out by the middle of the first semester of an online course. By the end of the first course, learners generally feel comfortable maneuvering around the virtual classroom and have increased comfort and skill in working on the computer.

7. How does this "learning curve" affect the learner's ability to complete/succeed in the first online course?

7. A steep "learning curve" hampers students' ability to succeed in their first online course. It is difficult to learn both new technology and new content at the same time. Orientation to the technology prior to the beginning the course can help make students' learning curve less steep.

8. What type of changes should learners expect as they make the transition to online learning?

8. In online learning, faculty members move from the traditional role as knowledge providers to the role of facilitators of learning. Students have a much more active role in their own learning. Since information is shared electronically and student-faculty interaction is limited by time and space, students' ability to work independently and to be accountable for completion of required readings is imperative. Carefully developed critical thinking activities can be planned to ensure group learning and personal support using a combination of synchronous and asynchronous communication allowing students to apply the information presented in the required readings. Students have to think critically and judge information for themselves. E-learning allows interactivity; thus, the learner need not be a passive recipient of knowledge. This individualization of learning, increased interactivity, and collaboration with others adds to the shift of education from being largely teacher-centered to student-centered, something educational researchers have been advocating for years. In the new learning paradigm, the absence of a highly structured experience may be disconcerting and stressful since it requires that students change their attitudes and beliefs about learning.

9. What are the norms for online participation?

9. Norms for the online classroom need to be established early to avoid confusion and misunderstanding. Norms include using basic netiquette, active participation in online classroom (either discussion board or chat room), and respecting privacy and confidentiality. These norms help to establish and maintain a sense of community.

Netiquette includes using students' names, respecting the views of others, avoiding hostile remarks, and judicious use of humor. Students unfamiliar with netiquette should be referred to one of the many Internet sites on netiquette for further information.

The syllabus should clarify expectations for active participation in the online classroom. It is important to lay out expectations early. Specify if you want students to logon a specific number of times per week or to check e-mail frequently to avoid confusion and frustration from differing expectations. Things go much more smoothly when everyone knows the expectations. Making participation a significant portion of the course grade also helps to motivate participation and encourage students to provide substantive information in their postings.

Participation in the online classroom is critical for active learning and successful achievement of learning outcomes. Learners in online courses often identify critical reflection as secondary benefit to participation in an asynchronous discussion board. Their reflection is an active, thoughtful, and intentional consideration of the learning material that provides opportunities for additional insights to enhance the learning experience.

Since participation in e-learning courses is often text-based using threaded discussions, students should be oriented to posting relevant comments that are substantive in nature and threading comments appropriately to avoid confusion on the discussion board.

Establishing a sense of community also is necessary to overcome the barriers of distance and technology, and the lack of visual cues. Introduction of class members and posting of pictures helps the establishment of a sense of community and familiarity. A supportive environment where participation of all group members is encouraged and responses are acknowledged helps to maintain the sense of community throughout the course.

10. What are the best ways to orient learners to the norms of new roles in e-learning?

10. Students should be informed of the changes in learning and the new roles of faculty and students at the beginning of the course. Faculty role modeling new norms provides guidance in adapting to the changes. Some discomfort should be expected as students adapt to the new roles. Learners are initially uncomfortable and unhappy with their increased responsibility for learning and change in faculty role; however, by the end of the first online course students are satisfied with their personal growth and are appreciative of the active role that they played in their own learning.

11. How do I deal with the initial student discomfort with new learning roles?

11. Give frequent, supportive feedback to students experiencing discomfort with the new learning roles. Encouragement is crucial to help students through the adjustment period. Faculty role modeling of the appropriate norms assists with the transition process. Referral to student mentors who have successfully completed an online course may also be helpful. These student mentors can provide tips to help new students to be successful.

12. When should I expect students to logon for the first time?

12. Generally students will not logon until sometime during the first week of classes, unless instructed to do otherwise. Some faculty members send students a welcome letter one to two weeks before the start of classes encouraging students to logon the week before classes start. This allows students to discover any technology glitches before the semester begins and keeps them from falling behind. Logging on early also helps students to be organized and ready to go when the semester officially begins.

13. How can I "get students to class" the first week and have them ready to learn?

13. Encourage students both in an introductory letter before the semester begins and via e-mail or the announcements section of the course to logon early and often. Without an introductory letter telling students the date they need to first logon and giving them instructions on how to logon, getting students to class the first week will occur later rather than sooner. Students new to e-learning may think that they can logon "anytime the first week or so," when you expect them to logon the first day of the week and complete an assignment by day four or five of that week. An introductory letter can avoid this misunderstanding and provide a smooth beginning to the course.

It is also crucial that faculty members participate actively during the first week of the course or module. Faculty should logon multiple times the first week to provide rich, rapid feedback to students logging on for the first time. Rapid feedback provides a positive experience for students, increases their engagement in the course, and this yields benefits as the course continues.

RESOURCES

Mueller, C. L. (2001). *Master's in nursing students' experiences in a virtual classroom on the Internet.* Unpublished doctoral dissertation.

Mueller, C. L., & Billings, D. M. (2000). Focus on the learner. In J. Novotny (Ed.), *Distance education in nursing* (pp. 65–84). New York: Springer.

Norton, B. (1998). From teaching to learning: Theoretical foundations. In D. M. Billings & J. A. Halstead (Eds.), *Teaching in nursing: A guide for faculty* (pp. 211–245). Philadelphia: Saunders.

Palloff, R. M., & Pratt, K. (2001). *Lessons from the cyberspace classroom: The realities of on-line teaching.* San Francisco: Jossey-Bass.

Simpson, O. (2000). *Supporting students in open and distance learning.* Sterling, VA: Stylus Publishing.

Section 6:
Designing Courses and Modules

E-learning courses are not mapped out in three-hour weekly class sessions for a 15-week semester, a one-hour staff development mandatory class, or a three-day continuing education conference—they are available on time and just-in-time. As you design e-courses, you will be thinking about content and course sequence in new ways. You will be using course-planning tools such as storyboards and course plans to organize and sequence learning. Because e-courses use multimedia, you must give attention to visual and graphic layout, course design, and Web interface functionality. In this unit you will learn about the additional expertise you will need to design courses, how to coordinate a course design team, and receive "tips" for making the course attractive and easy to use.

Chapter 18: Where Do I Start to Develop a Web Course?

1. I have just learned I am going to teach a course on the Web. Where do I start?

1. Start with getting course content together. Use traditional course material to help you with this. Prepare a table of contents or outline so you have an overview of the entire course and work from there. Use the class schedule to help. If you are thinking about using graphics, compile them now. Find time to work on the course. Look for sources of assistance, for example, a secretary, technical support staff, or someone outside the organization.

2. How should I organize content?

2. The course is no longer constrained by a weekly "semester" schedule. You can now organize the course in a way to facilitate learning! Begin with the table of contents, which is basically an outline of the course. Then break down the table of contents into units, modules, lessons, or weeks. Now, create learning activities that can be completed in a reasonable amount of time.

3. How do I organize course material for the best use by the learner?

3. Keep it simple. Use material you have used before and tested. This can be a big help when you are in a time crunch. Also, for each learning outcome, ask yourself "what learning activities will help students achieve this outcome"? (See Chapter 25 for more information.)

4. How can I organize the course so I have consistency in font and style across all content, units, modules, lessons, or weeks?

4. For the novice educator, I suggest using a Web editor such as Microsoft FrontPage® or Dreamweaver®. Both editors have templates called "wizards" or "styles" to help you keep consistent or this process could be done manually by selecting all of the material then changing the font and style to what you prefer. Once you are comfortable with the online environment, using "cascading style sheets" is the best way to organize and maintain consistency of font and style. (See Chapter 20.)

5. How can I design the course to keep my workload reasonable?

5. The first step in designing the course is to make a table of contents of what you are going to teach. Then branch off from that. You can either delete or add to the table of contents as you begin to design the course. Another time saver is to keep a list of questions learners ask repeatedly. Streamline your work by making a Web page of FAQs (Frequently Asked Questions). Another suggestion is to make a Resources Web page with links to documents or forms that learners will access often.

6. Can I put everything that I have taught in the classroom on the Web?

6. You could, but it will be too much information. I suggest that you modify content to make it easier for you and the learners to adjust. Highlight key points to begin with and expand on the material each time you teach the course.

Designing courses for the Web is different from developing "classroom" courses. Developing Web courses takes a lot of time so the key is to simplify course material into units, modules, lessons, or weeks.

7. I have a lot of handouts for the course. What is the best way to present them on the Web?

7. Linking documents to the course is usually the best choice because it saves space and time. However, be sure learners will have the appropriate software to open linked documents. For example, you have linked a Microsoft PowerPoint presentation; the user would have to have Microsoft PowerPoint Reader on the computer he/she is using in order to open it. You can convert Microsoft PowerPoint presentations into a Web format, but several files are made, which can make it confusing for both the educator and the user.

If you have handouts that are saved as text files, they can be easily converted to Rich Text Format (.rtf) and then inserted into a Web editor. If you have really complicated word processing documents, you may want to make a Web page of links and link to the document. Be sure that you are using original works for handouts or secure appropriate permissions.

8. Can I just type my lectures?

8. Yes, but that would be very boring for learners and what you want are dynamic learning experiences. Find a good textbook to provide background information, and then design learning activities to assist learners to apply the content.

9. Do you have suggestions for organizing multiple types of media when putting a Web-based course together?

9. First, gather all types of media (e.g., Microsoft PowerPoint, audio, video, and Web sites) you are thinking about using. Second, create a Web page that links to your media choices. Third, maintain the page to keep it up to date.

10. How should I pace assignments and due dates?

10. Pacing assignments can be done just as in a classroom situation. Consider the work involved for the leaner and spread assignments over a reasonable time frame. Remember, learners will be doing preparation (e.g., reading, writing, drafts, thinking) prior to completing the assignment, and this will entail considerable time.

11. How much time will it take to complete developing a Web course?

11. Time to complete course development varies. The time will depend on how the course is developed and in what electronic format such as the syllabus, tests, and handouts. If learning activities are already well developed

from a classroom course this will decrease the course development time. Also, you will need to consider your own technical skills and how easily you can do this yourself. Many institutions provide approximately six weeks (spread over time) to develop a 3 credit or 45 contact hour course.

12. What form do my files need to be in to get uploaded and look just as I intend them to?

12. First of all there is no word processor file format that will look attractive as a Web page. Therefore, any file will need to be "tweaked" to make it look professional on the Internet. I believe the best format for forwarding files to be posted in online courses is Rich Text Format (.rtf). This format allows an educator to convert a word processing document into a Rich Text Format and then insert the document into a Web editor.

I also recommend that if you are a Microsoft Word user that you automatically insert Word documents into a Web editor. You will still need to "tweak" the documents, but you eliminate the step of converting files to Rich Text Format.

13. What is the best format for material to be presented on the Web?

13. All material used on the Web must be in HTML format. HTML is the programming language the Internet reads. If you use a Web editor to create pages, you will not need to know this language; the editor will do it for you.

14. How do I get course material posted to a Web site?

14. Unless you are skilled in Web programming and have access to the institution's Web server, you will need technical assistance. Find out who the technical personnel are at the institution. There will be a person(s) to whom you will send finished Web-ready files. That person(s) will get those files on the Web site.

15. Where can I find ideas for the best layout for the course?

15. Surf the Internet and see what other educators have done. Jot down ideas of things you liked and didn't like about some of the courses and the way content is organized. Enroll in online courses to experience what works or does not. You can also go to some of the Web course software Web sites to try out the software. Some companies will let you set up a Web course for free; others may have a fee (see Chapter 10).

16. How can I make the Web course inviting, not messy or too complex?

16. Find assistance within your work setting! Find out who knows how to program Web pages and enlist that person to help you. A Web programmer is a must and can make the Web course look dynamic. If you cannot find such a person, then use a Web editor, such as Front Page. Web editors are easy to use and you do not need to know

17. *How do learners get access to yet maintain the confidentiality of documents such as clinical evaluations?*

18. *What are some ways to make a Web course more personal for users?*

19. *How can I be sure instructions about course activities, expectations, and assignments are clear to users?*

20. *How can I be more efficient in developing a Web course?*

21. *Do I need to create the entire course all at one time?*

programming. Web editors have templates that simplify how to make the course look attractive.

17. Faculty can use a well-secured Web course software package. These software packages have been designed to assure users that confidentiality will be maintained for evaluations, exams, and course data.

18. A welcome page is always a nice way to introduce yourself to learners and let them know a little bit about you. Adding a picture of yourself to the welcome page or somewhere within the Web course can also make you more real to users. You can also use different backgrounds, fonts, and graphics that appeal to you and at the same time maintain a professional image.

19. Instructions need to be explained simply but thoroughly for the person who has never used a computer or taken a Web course. I suggest that instructions or a "read me first" document be made available to learners before class begins. After all instructions are written, you can e-mail them to learners. If learners still do not understand, give them a support staff's telephone number who is able to help them one-on-one with a specific area. Or make yourself available to the first time students through virtual office hours or on the telephone.

20. One way to be more efficient is to use templates. Decide how you want your Web pages to look; for example, font, background, and graphics (see Chapter 20). Once you have a template in place your work will be easier. Use an HTML editor such as Microsoft FrontPage, which is similar to a word processor and helps keep pages looking the same.

21. No, break the Web course into smaller portions. To begin, complete only a basic course. Then build on the course each time it is offered. Continue making the course more dynamic by adding or refining the learning activities.

RESOURCES

Gookin, D. (1999). *Word 2000 for Windows for dummies*. New York: Hungry Minds, Inc.

Parker, E. (1999). *The complete idiot's guide to Microsoft FrontPage 2000*. Indianapolis, IN: Queue.

Chapter 19: *Storyboards and Course Plans*

1. What is the difference between a storyboard and a course plan?

1. A storyboard is a visual representation of the components of an online course. A good storyboard provides a roadmap that you can follow to reach the successful conclusion of course development. It is the map from where you start to your destination.

A course plan is a document that helps you design a course, outlining the components of the course content, identifying the learning outcomes, the learning and teaching strategies, the assessment and evaluation strategies, and mapping the visual components that will enhance the content.

2. I know my subject matter/I've been teaching for a long time/I've taught this course many times in the classroom, I simply need to move it online. Why do I need a course plan or storyboard?

2. There may be many reasons for planning or storyboarding a course, whether it's one that has been taught numerous times, or a fresh idea that you are developing for the first offering.

Course planning and storyboarding allow you the opportunity to take a fresh look at the subject matter, consider peer and student evaluations, and try new teaching and learning strategies. Course planning may provide you the opportunity to move from an instructor-centric approach ("the sage on the stage") to a learner-centric approach (with the faculty as the "guide on the side").

E-learning, particularly Web-based learning, is valuable because it allows learners multiple channels or pathways to instruction. In many cases, it allows learners to traverse the content in a nonlinear fashion. Storyboarding a course allows you to lay out various channels and determine multiple entry points to specific topics and instructional segments, or to determine those areas where the learner should be guided to work in a linear fashion for some specified period of time or purpose.

3. What do I need to use to create a storyboard and a course plan?

3. Neither storyboards or course plans have to be created with a particular tool. Often, a designer's choice of creation tools depends upon his/her preferred learning and teaching style, time available for planning, expertise in teaching in this particular learning environment, length of learning module, and whether the course is a new course or the redesign of an existing course.

You can write a textual narrative, or create a flowchart or a concept map. If you prefer the low-tech method, use 3x5 or 4x6 index cards that you can rearrange and annotate as you plan the course.

4. Are there certain components that you regard as essential elements in a storyboard for the course?

4. A storyboard should provide a visual representation of the elements of a page within the course. It should identify which components you will include and where they should be located in the course. The storyboard should also identify the formatting and attributes of each element (see Figure 1).

Figure 1. *Storyboard*

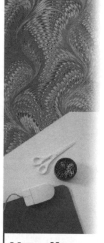

INSTRUCTIONAL SEGMENT TITLE
centered, Verdana, 14pt, bold, all caps

Body text, left-aligned, Verdana, 12pt

Body text, left-aligned, Verdana, 12pt

Heading left-aligned, Verdana, 12pt, bold

This is a new section, denoted by the heading to the left. If hyperlinks are included, the link should be worked into the text. For example, see <u>more information</u> on penguins.

 Page Back

 Page Forward

Additional notations can be made in either textual or visual format. For example: keep the "page back" and "page forward" notations on each sub-page. For the first page, the "page back" can be removed; for the last page, the "page forward" can be removed.

5. So you're saying that a storyboard is like a generic page with most, if not all, of the page elements included so that I can refer to it during development to keep pages consistent. How does that differ from a course planning document?

5. The storyboard is about how the page looks. The course plan is concerned more with what the content includes.

6. Which elements should I make sure to include in a course planning document?

6. I recommend that you begin with the *description* of the learning segment. This will provide the overview of what the course entails.

You should also include the *learning objectives*. Learning objectives are also referred to as *course competencies* or *learning outcomes*. They provide the learner with a concrete description of what he/she should have mastered upon the successful conclusion of the learning experience. Too often objectives are written in vague terms that do not provide either the learner or the instructor with details of what learning should occur. Learning objectives that are written as concrete, measurable outcomes provide both the instructor and learner with the basis for evaluation and assessment.

Based upon the learning objectives that you have specified, begin to identify the *learning activities* that the learners should participate in. Both you and the learners will find it helpful to match learning activities with specific learning objectives. This will ensure that you have included the necessary learning activities to enable the learner to meet the learning outcomes. Be sure to identify several activities in order to address the variety of learning styles that learners will bring to the course.

In addition to learning activities, identify the *teaching strategies* that you will use in the course. The richness of the Web as a learning environment allows you to employ a variety of strategies including text-based lectures, audio/video, images, individual and group projects, discussion, and many others. Additional course planning elements should include notation of where tables, figures, graphics, and images can be used to enhance the learning content, and references and resources for further exploration of topics for both you and the learner.

In the planning document, be sure to include *assessment and evaluation strategies*. Identify ways that you can assess the student learning in this environment where you often never see students.

RESOURCES

Buhmann, J. (2000). *Designing Web pages and integrating media. On-line course: Teaching & evaluation.* Indianapolis: Indiana University School of Nursing, Lifelong Learning.

Dell, D. (2000). *Instructional teams. On-line course: Getting started.* Indianapolis: Indiana University School of Nursing, Lifelong Learning.

Hollingsworth, C. D. (2000). *Making effective presentations/Using color effectively.* Indiana University Purdue University Indianapolis (IUPUI) Web site:
http://www.iupui.edu/~webtrain/tutorials/effective_visual_aids.htm

Chapter 20: *Layout, Fonts, Colors, Graphics*

1. *I need to start at the beginning . . . what do you mean by layout, fonts, colors, and graphics?*

1. *Layout* is the term used to describe how elements such as text, figures, tables, and images fit on a page or screen. Designers usually think of layout in terms of a grid that gives each element its own space on a page or screen. Figure 1 shows a sample grid layout that might be used for a page having a title, a left and a right margin, and a center area for text. The grid lines themselves are visible only to the designers and don't display on the page or screen, leaving only the appearance of a well-spaced page.

Figure 1. *Sample Grid Layout*

TITLE		
	Textual content goes in this middle space. Notice that as you write content and the text "grows" that it gives the appearance of both a left and a right margin.	

Fonts define the style and shape of letters. Some letters have "feet" at the bottom, as if to support the letters. Serif fonts have "feet" and are the "traditional" font faces. Other letters are clean, without "feet;" these are sans-serif fonts.

Pages and screens are often described as having white space, black space, and gray space. White space is the open area; gray space is the area composed of text; and black space is the space used by images. White, black, and gray spaces are considered a part of the page layout since they are defining the type of element on a page or screen. Colors, on the other hand, can be divided into two components: background and foreground. Background is the "wallpaper" or "paint" on which all other page or screen elements "sit." Foreground is the text and image elements of the page or screen.

2. *Is there an ideal layout for an online course?*

2. Not necessarily. It is important to develop a layout that makes it easy for learners to locate any information they may need. The use of white space and a consistent use of spacing and layout will make it easy for the reader to scan for information.

All written materials, but particularly online materials, should pass the "squint test"—after developing a section of material sit back and squint—the purpose is not to read the text, but to see that there is balance and consistent amounts of spacing between sections and headings and to determine that even without reading you would be able to correctly identify specific components in the materials because of their size, shape, placement, and coloration.

3. What is the best layout and design tip you can give me?

3. For many Web and instructional designers who work with online instructional materials, the layout and design mantra should be "tables are my friend." By using a table to assist with the layout of your content, you can effectively control left and right margins easily (see Figure 1). Too often, text on Web pages is allowed to abut the margin, leaving the content too close to the edges of the browser window to be easily read. Using a table, with the left and right columns empty and no borders on the table, gives the visual appearance of a well-designed page with ample margins.

One layout methodology that has been used with great success in both print and electronic publications is Information Mapping®

4. What is Information Mapping®?

4. Information Mapping® (imap) is a methodology that was developed to organize and manage information. It has been used successfully throughout Europe for both print and online information, and is a preferred style for educational, promotional, organizational, and commercial documentation around the world.

Using the imap methodology, content is organized by "chunking" text into logical units. The layout of documents has "out-dented" headings—rather than the headings being aligned on the left margin with the text, headings are in a "column" to the left of the text. This separates the headings from the body of information. The Information Mapping® format improves the reader's ability to easily locate pertinent material by quickly scanning a page of text. Imap methodology is documented on the Web site **http://www.imap.dk/imapexample.htm**. Compare the example of a business document written in a traditional business format with that same document laid out using the information mapping methodology.

5. Are certain font choices easier to read online than others?

5. As mentioned above, fonts are divided into two types: serif and sans serif. Serif fonts are those "traditional" fonts where letters such as r, f, and h have "feet" that appear to give the letters stability. Times Roman and

Courier are common examples of serif font faces. Sans serif fonts are "clean," without "feet." Arial and Helvetica are two common examples. Verdana is a sans serif font face that was developed specifically for online use. Letters in the Verdana font are spaced wider, leaving text written in this font crisp and easy to read.

In general, sans serif fonts are easier to read online, while serif fonts should be used for print materials.

Examples:

This sentence is written in Times Roman (a traditional serif font).

This sentence is written in Verdana (a sans serif font developed specifically for online text).

Even though both of the preceding example sentences are written using the same font size, note the difference in size. Think how much less strain it would place on your eyes to read the Verdana font, especially online, over a lengthy period of time.

6. Are there certain fonts that I should avoid using in online instructional materials?

6. There are thousands of font faces available today (and more being developed every day!). Many course developers and authors, in an effort to be unique, consider using a variety of stylistic fonts in their work. Authors should always keep in mind that fonts reside on individual computers. This means that when an author designs text to appear a particular way, if that specific font isn't installed on the reader's computer then the text written using that font face can't be displayed as the designer intended it.

If you create a document using a font face called Bohemian, but I don't have that specific font installed on my computer, then my computer will choose one of the installed fonts that it "thinks" may be close to Bohemian and show the text to me using that alternate. Sometimes those substitutions can lead to very strange or difficult to read text.

Although we each want to be creative, when it comes to font choices, you should stick with the standards that are likely to be installed on most computers. If you want a sans serif font, consider using Verdana, Arial, or Helvetica. The serif font choices would include Times Roman, Schoolbook, Garamond, or Courier.

7. *Since the stylistic fonts might not display correctly on the reader's computer, how can I show creativity by using only a mix of those standards you referred to above?*

7. Keep in mind that even creativity should have a purpose beyond just being "different" or "exciting." Everything you include on a Web page should have purpose and meaning. This helps readers orient themselves in the material and helps them focus on the content rather than the design of the instructional materials.

You should restrict the number of fonts within a document or page to no more than three. Ideally, you should use a single font face for all of the text, including headings (remember you can use formatting and/or color for emphasis). If you really feel strongly that you want to use multiple font faces, choose one to use for all the body text, and a different one to use for all headings.

An exception to the "rule of three" is when you are writing instructions, for example, in working with a computer. In addition to the font faces you use for text and headings, you may need to also choose a different font or formatting to indicate commands the learner should type exactly as indicated, information that the learner must supply, menu selections, or labels on buttons. See Figure 2 for an example of how you might choose to format instructions on adding a header to a word processing document.

Figure 2. *Format for Instructions*

> **To add a header to a Word document:**
>
> 1. From the menu, choose, VIEW : Header and Footer.
> 2. In the box, type: *Conversations in E-Learning*.
> 3. After you've finished typing, click the Close button.

8. *In my work, I use a lot of special symbols, "Wingding" and "Symbol" characters and foreign letters. I can't use the standard font faces for those—what should I do?*

8. You're absolutely correct that the standard fonts will not work in those situations. Furthermore, you can't take a chance that the reader might not have the foreign language, "Symbol" or "Wingding" fonts installed, leaving the possibility that the meaning of the text could be radically altered. In these situations, your best option is to create a graphic that displays the special characters you need.

All graphics applications including Adobe Photoshop®, Microsoft Image Composer®, and Paint Shop Pro®, allow you to type text using any font face you choose from your computer. Then you can choose any colors or formatting that you want applied to the text. Some applications also allow you to add special effects such as three-dimension, spotlighting, and distortions. After you have completed formatting the text, you can save the text, with its special effects and colors, as an image (make sure that your graphics application allows you to save in either gif or jpeg formats—which I discuss below—so that they're Web-readable). When you insert the image into your Web page, it's treated as any other image or photograph would be, meaning that it doesn't matter what fonts you or the reader have available, since it is treated the same as any other photograph or graphic would be treated.

9. What size font should I use?

9. There is no "hard and fast" rule that I can give you; the best response is to avoid extremes and to be consistent. The way that the fonts display on a computer depends upon the monitor resolution that the reader has chosen for his/her computer. This means that something that appears small on your computer monitor could well appear VERY small on someone else's monitor, or vice versa.

In general, you should use headings that are about 14-point and body text that is about 12-point. I would not recommend that you ever use fonts less than 10-point (unless it's a "footer" type of information that you don't really expect anyone to read—but even then, if it's important enough that you need to include it, it must be large enough for the reader to be able to easily read). You can sometimes use 18-point size for a main title, but generally anything larger than that is extreme.

If you use a visual editor, such as FrontPage® or Dreamweaver®, you may see an option on the toolbar for styles. Included in the choices are H1, H2, H3, and so on. These are Hypertext Mark-up Language (HTML) codes that correspond roughly to font sizes: an H1 heading is about a 14-point size, while an H2 is about 12-point. However, you should use heading tags only for titles and headings because they also include spacing that would not be appropriate for most content text. Use normal or 12-point for most body text.

145

10. *How do I make effective color choices when designing online materials?*

10. Color choice can be one of the most difficult decisions to make when designing online materials (or any other publication) because preferences for colors are so highly personal and subjective. However, there are four basic rules that you are encouraged to consider when designing online materials:

1. Understand that there is a difference between printed and displayed colors.

2. Understand the basic components of color design.

3. Ensure that there is sufficient contrast between the foreground and background elements of your page.

4. Use effective color combinations.

11. *I've noticed that the colors on printed pages don't look like they appear on a Web page. Why?*

11. Colors displayed through a computer are blends of red, green, and blue (RGB). Computers display color by "pushing" light through the screen—the light is within the monitor.

Print colors are blends of cyan, yellow, magenta, and black (CMYK). The colors are blended and reflected from the color of the page they are printed on.

12. *What are the basic elements of color design that I should be aware of?*

12. Color design is based on the "color wheel" (You can find an example of the color wheel online at **http://www.iupui.edu/~webtrain/color_wheel.jpg**) REMEMBER—displayed color appears differently than print color, so use the wheel as a "rule of thumb" rather than an absolute measure of colors).

Primary colors (yellow, magenta, and cyan) are the colors on the outside of the wheel. Secondary colors (red, green, and blue) are the colors on the inside of the wheel. Cool colors (blues and greens) appear to recede from the user and should, therefore, be used for background coloration. Warm colors (reds, yellows, and oranges) appear to approach the user and should, therefore, be used for foreground coloration. (Foreground includes anything placed on the background, such as text, graphics, and figures.)

A good contrast of colors provides warmth, energy, clarity, and sharpness to pages. However, too much contrast introduces confusion and is overwhelming.

There are national, cultural, religious, and holiday implications with color choices as well. You can most likely think of some color combinations yourself that cause you to think or feel certain ways. When it comes to color choices, knowledge of the audience should help guide you in the decisions you make.

The most important element of color design that should be relied upon is "less is more"—especially when you are considering backgrounds. Always remember that the content should be the most prominent—not the colors or designs you chose to use.

13. Speaking of backgrounds, what are some guidelines on using patterned or print "wallpaper" on Web pages?

13. Some designers like to use print or patterned background on Web pages. The most important thing to remember is that any background should not compete with content (the foreground). You should look for wallpapers with subtle patterns and those where the contrast is decreased so that the patterns and colors are muted.

One effective choice is to use wallpaper that appears as a border on the left side of the page. This option gives you some flexibility in design and allows your personality to show, yet allows the area of the page where the content will be to remain "clean."

14. What does sufficient contrast between foreground and background mean?

14. Black print on white paper has survived the test of time in print publications—even when color was readily available. One of the reasons for this is because that specific combination provides sufficient contrast to be easily read. One way to ensure enough contrast is to remember to use cool colors for backgrounds and warm colors for foreground elements.

You will have the greatest contrast of colors when you use pairs of primary colors (If you need a refresher on color combinations, review the color wheel at **http://www.iupui.edu/~Webtrain/Graphics/Tutorials/color_wheel.jpg**). Choosing complementary contrasting pairs is easy when you remember to always choose a secondary color and the primary color that falls opposite it on the color wheel. One of the more effective color combinations is yellow on blue.

15. Have you ever heard (or said): "I've got to find some graphics to break up all the text on this page"?

15. Images should be used to explain and enhance text, not simply used because you have too many words. Rather than approaching your project with "where can I stick a picture?" instead approach it with "will a diagram, chart, photograph, or visual representation make this idea or concept more clear and less ambiguous?"

16. GIF? JPEG? What do they mean?! You might as well be talking ABC and XYZ!

16. Graphics Interchange Format (GIF) and Joint Photographic Experts Group (JPEG) are two image formats that are readable by Web browsers. Image files can be very large files, even when the photograph or graphic itself isn't. Large files mean slow download times; and if the download time is considered excessive by the person attempting to view the page, he/she will likely leave before ever reading the content. Both GIF and JPEG formats are compression applications, meaning that correctly used they can decrease (often dramatically) the size of the image file with little or no loss of quality.

JPEG is a *lossy* compression format. Lossy compression means that it actually removes bits of color in order to reduce the file size. JPEG is the format you should use when you want to put a photographic image on the Web. Photographs (and other images that have a lot of gradient, blended colors) are composed of millions of colors. JPEG removes colors—most of which our eyes can't see—to decrease the number of colors in the image, thus reducing the size of the file.

GIF's compression format works differently—it records a "marker" for each unique color it encounters in the graphic. If it encounters a color for which it already has a marker, it ignores that color. This is why GIF is the appropriate format for graphics that have large blocks of solid colors, such as those bullets, bars, cubes, arrows, and clipart that have solid, rather than blended colors.

17. I've also heard of PNG and ART. You didn't mention them. What are they?

17. Portable Network Graphics (PNG) is an emerging Web image format. Some applications are beginning to have PNG as an option, but until it becomes more widely available, I would stick with GIF or JPEG.

ART is a proprietary image format created and used by America Online™. It is not a standard Web-readable format and is only used by AOL. In fact, if you try to save an image you find while using AOL, it will automatically save as an ART file—rendering it unviewable by most Web users. So, if you find an ART image that you want to use, you will need to also have available an image application that will read that specific format so that it can be converted—meaning an AOL browser. With the huge number and vast amount of styles of images that are readily available, I strongly recommend that you avoid ART files.

18. How do I find images to use in instructional materials?

18. The choices for locating images are as varied as the images themselves. You can purchase stock photography and clip art collections at any retail store that sells computer applications. Some textbook publishers also grant purchasers of their textbooks access to online resources. One of the most common locations for Web images, though, is the Web itself. Some of the search engines and directories, such as Yahoo, have an image category.

Be aware that searching the Web for images can often be a taxing experience. You will stumble upon a few great resources while encountering numerous sites containing less than ideal resources. Be aware, also, that simply searching for "images" or "photographs" may result in locating sites containing obscene or pornographic images. Quite often, your best choice for locating images is to talk to colleagues who can identify sites that they have found useful.

19. How do I decide which graphics to use?

19. Remember that learners each approach learning situations from very individual backgrounds. What looks like a coffee mug to you may look like a coffee cup to me. The same four-legged animal may be a mule, a donkey, a horse, a pony, or a stallion to five different individuals, depending upon their background and history. Keep things simple and unambiguous. Be sure that text and graphics complement one another and don't leave learners confused or developing knowledge on misconceptions.

20. I'm concerned about infringing the copyright of images that I find and want to use. How do I address that?

20. Another chapter in this book discusses copyright issues. However, from the point of using images, I would recommend that you read through the sites. Almost all sites will tell you somewhere whether you are free to use the images and under what circumstances. Just remember that everything has a copyright holder, whether it is stated or not. When in doubt, get permission or find another source.

21. I'm the teacher/ educator/content expert. Do I really need to know all of this?

21. Education—particularly online education—has long since passed the time when a single individual could effectively and efficiently take a course from concept through design, development, delivery, and maintenance. Effective online instructional design requires the skill-sets of a team of professionals. The individuals involved and their roles are identified in Table 1.

Table 1. *Online Instructional Design Team*

Member	Role
Educator	Subject matter expert, learning facilitator, guide, coach, mentor
Instructional Designer	Advises regarding content sequence, delivery, learning activities, pedagogical principles
Librarian	Assists with locating online and library resources; develops Web site resources page
Learning Resources Coordinator	Assists with locating instructional resources/software
Multimedia Developer	Integrates multimedia into course; develops tutorials using multimedia
Webmaster/File Server and LAN Manager	Manages Web site; posts course to Web site; maintains links to course and resources; maintains network
Videoconferencing Coordinator	Designs course for TV delivery; manages TV classroom; facilitates reception sites
Video Producer	Produces videotape, digital video, instructional pieces
Copyright Specialist	Advises about copyright and intellectual property, contract, copyright clearance
Technical Transfer Specialist	Works with faculty to find commercial opportunities for course materials and develops royalty agreements
Bookstore Manager	Devises mechanisms for students at a distance (not on campus) to order books, course materials, learning resources, computer hardware, software
Student Mentor	Student who has been through course who can provide advice and support to students who need support as they learn to use new course delivery mechanisms
Teaching Assistant	Assists faculty with teaching the class; provides additional support to students needing tutoring
Technical Support Personnel	Available to assist students and faculty with technical problems or course delivery; orients students and faculty to the use of the technology being used to deliver the course
Assessment/Evaluation Specialist	Designs evaluation plans for course, faculty, and program
Graphic Designer	Integrates graphics into course/media; ensures visual balance, color comparability, aesthetic quality
Programmer	Uses computer languages, HTML, and authoring software to develop multimedia programs

RESOURCES

Buhmann, J. (2000). *Designing Web pages and integrating media. Online course: Teaching & evaluation.* Indianapolis: Indiana University School of Nursing, Lifelong Learning.

Dell, D. (2000). *Instructional teams. Online course: Getting started.* Indianapolis: Indiana University School of Nursing, Lifelong Learning.

Hollingsworth, C. D. (2000). *Making effective presentations / Using color effectively.* http://www.iupui.edu/~Webtrain/tutorials/effective_visual_aids.htm

Section 7:
The Online Learning Community

Learning is a social activity, and learning in the health professions involves interaction with faculty, other learners, experts, health professionals, and clients. The online learning community is the place in the Web course where all can come together to learn, to acquire professional values, become socialized to the profession, collaborate, conduct service learning projects, or prepare for real-world practice. Being a member of an online learning community requires a commitment to norms of behavior in which participants assume responsibility for learning, demonstrate respect for members of the community, engage in open and honest exchange of information, and participate in a timely manner. The role of the course educator-facilitator is to motivate, guide, and manage the community to achieve its goals. The authors of the chapters in this unit will help you establish a learning community and give you pointers about how to manage it for success.

Chapter 21: *The Online Learning Community*

1. What is an online community?

1. An online community is a collage of information, resources, activities, learning objectives, multimedia elements, and people connected and engaged in learning activities. The online learning community may use asynchronous and/or synchronous communications in an electronic environment. The community can include a wide range of learning activities and informational sources and linkages. Constituents of the online learning community include students and faculty as well as multi-disciplinary partners, clients, and support personnel.

2. How do I form a community?

2. An online learning community is formed first by establishing and ensuring the quality and reliability of the foundation for the community. There are several elements needed for the initial formation and maintenance of the online learning community. Elements include student and faculty support and connectedness to the online community, development of instructional materials, reliable and accessible technology infrastructure, and an evaluation and assessment plan. In considering all of these elements, there must be adherence to educational practices for online teaching.

3. What can educators do to facilitate the formation of a sense of community in an online class?

3. Educators can use a wide continuum of asynchronous and synchronous communication techniques and learning activities to facilitate the sense of community in an online class. An initial orientation is a good strategy. Other methods of keeping the group together include updating messages often, summarizing group and/or individual work, and asking questions and providing answers. Prompt and meaningful feedback, ideally within 24 hours, improves learning and connectedness. Student interaction with faculty and other students can be facilitated through numerous avenues, including voice-mail, e-mail, discussion boards, chat rooms, and videoconferencing. Teaching strategies focused on engagement and meaningful tasks also facilitate a sense of community in the online class. An example might be a Web-quest directing students to particular Web sites and resources for specific outcomes culminating in online discussions. The educator role of facilitator versus "sage on the stage" is often more conducive to community building in the online learning community.

4. What are the students' responsibilities in the online learning community?

4. Students are responsible for active and timely participation in the online learning community. Student interaction with faculty and other constituents of the community is an essential characteristic for community development and success. Students are also responsible for demonstrating the values and ethics of professional networking in the online learning community. The values are often illustrated through the public nature of the discussion board and/or forum postings to the entire community.

5. How do I overcome the sense of isolation?

5. A variety of asynchronous and/or synchronous communications and teaching strategies can be used to help overcome the sense of isolation that can occur in the online learning community. Advising and self-assessment prior to the online experience can help determine learner suitability and preference for online instructional delivery. An orientation to the online learning environment can facilitate a sense of community prior to the class as well as at the beginning of the class. Learners as well as educators should have ongoing technical support. Faculty need to provide prompt and meaningful feedback through a variety of electronic methods, such as e-mail, forum participation and facilitation, group messages, virtual office hours, and telephone calls. Other strategies that can decrease the sense of isolation may include the posting of digital photos of class participants, having students develop their own home pages in the course, or having scheduled chat times or videoconference sessions, if this technology is available.

6. How do I deal with nonverbal cues (lack of visual cues)?

6. The inclusion of netiquette in the student's and faculty's initial orientation to the online learning community is a good beginning in dealing with the lack of visual cues in many distance learning programs. This orientation can include some tips and ideas for enhancing professional networking and communication through often a primarily text based media. For example, use upper and lower case words rather than solely upper case, which implies shouting or anger in an e-mail message and/or forum posting. Timely clarification is also a good method to deal with nonverbal cues. A promptly mailed individual e-mail message may provide clarification of written cues. Likewise, a telephone call may help to resolve an issue.

7. How is the online community different from the classroom community?

7. The most obvious difference between the classroom and online community is the environmental setting. In the classroom setting the physical presence of other learners creates a sense of belonging to a community. The educator's presence can create a sense of security, even authority. Most educators have been oriented to and socialized into a traditional classroom setting that allows for face-to-face contact and verbal interactions. The non-verbal messages are equally as important in the classroom setting. Students depend on cues to follow the sequence of dialogue and determine their responses. Educators depend on cues to make decisions about the flow of content and discussions. The classroom environment allows for immediate answers to questions, spontaneity, and closure on discussion topics.

8. What can be done in the online community that cannot be done in the classroom?

8. The online community has a unique environment created by the individuals who are participating. Students cannot depend on the physical presence of other students or structure of the classroom to provide an atmosphere that requires time on task. Because of the lack of structure of the learning community, personal motivation and self-discipline are qualities that are required to work in an online environment. The upside of a non-structured learning environment is that participants can learn anywhere, any time. For most students and many faculty, the home is the learning environment. This atmosphere, although usually lacking face-to-face interactions, is comfortable and convenient. In contrast, travel to a university setting or a conference site can be inconvenient. Class and conference schedules may be inflexible or in conflict with work schedules. Convenience and flexibility have been reported in the literature as two prominent factors that make online learning preferable to the classroom setting.

The online educational environment allows for almost unlimited resources. While many classroom visuals have been incorporated into Web-based courses such as PowerPoint presentations, many opportunities are available to both faculty and students that enhance the exploration of ideas and concepts for all disciplines. Professional resources are only a link away.

Participation in learning activities has long been recognized as a key component of learning. Physical presence in a classroom does not indicate verbal or mental participation. In fact all may be seated in the classroom, but none of us know where the others really are. Another hallmark of online learning is participation. All participants must enter the virtual classroom armed with responses and resources. Required participation by every student makes online learning more valid in relation to student preparation, depth, and quality of assignments.

9. What can you do in the classroom that cannot be done in the online community?

9. In the classroom setting educators can manipulate certain aspects of the environment to support course content or unit outcomes. Visual aids of a variety of types have long been used to illustrate course content. For example, the blackboard, videotapes, current day PowerPoint presentations, and Web site demonstrations are available. While visual teaching support materials have been redesigned or transformed into Web delivery methods the difference between classroom and online delivery is that the classroom allows for interpersonal presence, immediate feedback and response. Responses are delayed in online learning due to a time lapse between posting and responding in asynchronous delivery.

RESOURCES

Cartwright, J. (2000). Lessons learned using asynchronous computer-mediated conferencing to facilitate group discussion. *Journal of Nursing Education, 39*(2), 87–90.

Landis, B. J., & Wainwright, M. (1996). Electronic education: Computer conferencing communication for distance learners. *Nurse Educator, 21*(2), 9–14.

Leasure, A.R., Davis, L., & Thievon, S. L. (2000). Comparison of student outcomes and preferences in a traditional versus World Wide Web-based baccalaureate nursing research course. *Journal of Nursing Education, 39*(4), 149–154.

Navarro, P., & Shoemaker, J. (2000). Performance and perceptions of distance learners in cyberspace. *American Journal of Distance Education, 14*(2), 15–35.

O'Malley, J., & McCraw, H. (1999). Student perceptions of distance learning, online learning and the traditional classroom. *Online Journal of Distance Learning Administration, 2*(4). Retrieved from **www.westga.edu**.

Ryan, M., Hodson Carlton, K., & Ali, N. S. (1999). Evaluation of traditional classroom methods versus course delivery via the World Wide Web. *Journal of Nursing Education, 38*(6), 272–277.

Vrasidas, C., & McIsaac, M. S. (1999). Factors influencing interaction in an on-line course. *The American Journal of Distance Education, 13*(3), 22–34.

Chapter 22: *Creating and Managing an Online Community*

1. How do I create an online community?

1. To create an online community, educators need to identify students, instructors, community leaders, and experts in a specific area, and develop partnerships with technology staff. There also needs to be assurance of the reliability of electronic tools such as software and courseware as well as the availability of links to Web sites in an online course. Faculty must have adequate skills to maintain dynamic interaction in this community and use designated criteria to evaluate qualities of online education.

2. What teaching strategies facilitate the formation of the community?

2. Educators can use a variety of teaching strategies including synchronous and asynchronous communication to promote a sense of community. The course or program can begin with having everyone introduce themselves and give some informal information about themselves. Warm up activities such as small group work or "round robin" postings give everyone a chance to participate and feel comfortable as the group forms.

As participants become more comfortable with sharing and revealing, other teaching strategies can include games, case study discussions, guest speaker participation, exploration of Web sites to substantiate posted information, debates, and group/individual responses. The community continues to form as everyone contributes and has a sense that their contributions are valued and contribute to course goals.

3. How do I maintain engagement in the online learning community?

3. To maintain engagement in the online community, different strategies are used. In course syllabi, points are assigned to participation and the criteria of active participation are described in details. For example, an individual response to a posted question should follow the stated criteria (for example: one page as a Word document and documented by three references). Posted questions by the instructor need to engage students in the learning process and critical thinking will be required to answer those questions. Specific practice-related assignments and the Web pages available in the course must be stimulating to students. Also due dates and designated times for the different assignments are stated in the course calendar for participation. Sometimes, an e-mail message or a phone call might motivate a student whose response is indicative of inactive participation.

4. How do I make the online community innovative?

4. A variety of activities are used to make the online community innovative. During a course, learners' comments and e-mail messages about the delivery of the online class are used in improving the course for the next term. Also trial and error is used to test different teaching strategies and positive experiences are re-used. Using a welcome video and streaming video for experts in a particular area are other methods. Assignments that require community engagement and multidisciplinary approaches are encouraged.

5. How do I continually update the online community?

5. Before the class starts, reexamine online course(s) including calendar, modules, assignments, etiquette, policies, and guidelines of the course. The availability of the different links to Web sites in the course should also be continually checked. Problems encountered in the previous course sequence are used to adjust the course for the current time period and positive experiences are repeated in the current course. Also, feedback from course evaluations and the nursing program's evaluation plan are used to update and improve courses continually.

6. How do I manage the participation in the online community?

6. I use a variety of strategies to manage students' participation in the online learning community. Design and development and/or editing of the course prior to actual implementation is an important first step. It helps to conceptualize the course into units or modules, which coincide with course outcomes and due dates. Content organization can create structure to help with course management, including facilitating and monitoring responses and follow-up. Once the course is implemented and students are enrolled, timely and constructive feedback to forum discussions helps ensure managerial success for the course. It is also essential that the reliability and quality of the infrastructure support are maintained and monitored for consistent service.

7. How do I manage due dates for assignments?

7. Due dates are managed by pre-planning, most advisably, prior to the implementation of the online course. Educators may decide to subtract points and/or completely delete a score for learning activities not completed by the due date.

In a course with large amounts of posting to the discussion board, it is helpful to set a date for discussion on a specific topic to end. Participants who have not contributed or who have additional points to make can do so with a private e-mail to course members or the faculty, so that all course members are not distracted by late contributions. A student who consistently cannot submit learning activities by the established due dates may be advised to reconsider his/her suitability for online learning.

8. How do I keep students motivated?

8. Providing engaging learning activities and communications can help keep students motivated in the online learning environment. Individual and community communications can provide continuity and a sense of purpose and connectedness through the progression of the online course. Assignments, which are relevant to practice and engaging, have the most success in keeping students motivated.

9. What are "lurkers" in an online community?

9. Lurkers are those who are present in the online community, but are not actively engaged in the activities. For example, the educator's course management statistics may indicate a "lurker" has been present in the online community; however, there is no posted evidence of the "lurker's" active engagement. The lurker is reading the postings of others, but is not posting communications and/or information.

10. How do I deal with lurkers?

10. I deal with lurkers in the online learning community with different strategies. Participation by established due dates can be required and evaluated with points and grades. Individual e-mail to the lurker can elicit individual problems and concerns while encouraging participation. A telephone call can also be a way to ascertain any reasons for the lack of participation.

11. What are "laggards" in an online community?

11. Laggards are those participants in the online community who are consistently late in responding to activities in the online course. For example, I post a due date for, perhaps, a discussion board entry by all students in the course, and the "laggard" posts an entry hours and days after the established due date.

12. How do I deal with laggards?

12. I deal with laggards by establishing guidelines for timely participation at the beginning of the online class. Ideally, an individual e-mail can be used to elicit an explanation about participation problems. A telephone call can also be used to determine reasons for this behavior. Points subtracted for late work is also a good way to deal with laggard behavior. If the behavior persists for an extended time, it may be good to advise the student to reconsider his/her suitability for online learning.

RESOURCES

Billings, D., Connors, H., & Skiba, D. (2001). Benchmarking best practices in Web-based nursing courses. *Advances in Nursing Science, 23*(3), 41–52.

Cartwright, J. (2000). Lessons learned using asynchronous computer-mediated conferencing to facilitate group discussion. *Journal of Nursing Education, 39*(2), 87–90.

Miller, M. (2001). The effect of e-mail messages on student participation in the asynchronous online course. *Online Journal of Distance Learning Administration, 4*(3). Retrieved from **www.westga.edu**

Chapter 23: The "Social Aspects" of the Online Learning Community

1. What is "social space" in the online community?

1. The social space in an online learning community can be conceptualized as the "student lounge," the "nurses' lounge," the "hallway," or the "canteen," in traditional educational settings. This is a space where the participants of the online community can meet for social comments separate from the comments specifically related to course activities. The social space may be within the one class community, such as a student discussion forum area or a chat room. It may also be a common area linked but established outside the particular course area for student and group social and informational discussions.

2. How do you establish "social space" in an online community?

2. To establish "social space" in an online community, faculty creates unmonitored online avenues for students to chat with each other without faculty's accessibility to these routes. These avenues might include chat rooms only for students—faculty cannot see chat logs of students, or setting up chat tools so that students can talk with each other outside the course. Also, faculty can set up a forum that is to be used only for sharing information not related to the business of the course—which both learners and educators can use. A community of students' link is another area where students can chat with each other, exchange ideas, and ventilate feelings without taking time off the course discussion.

3. How can students and faculty build social relationships within an online community?

3. Students and faculty build social relationships working collaboratively on learning activities through an entire spectrum of communication possibilities. Communication modes include telephone and teleconferencing sessions, asynchronous electronic mail messages, and discussion and forum areas. Other methods include the synchronous tools of chat sessions and videoconferencing, and occasional and/or planned face-to-face clinical visits and/or meetings. Social relationships develop from a range of individual and group interactions. This range of relationships may include frequent and timely feedback from the student(s), faculty facilitator/moderator, and other participants of the online course and linked communities and resources.

4. Whose responsibility is it to maintain social spaces?

4. It is the responsibility of all participants of the online learning community to maintain the availability of established social spaces. Just as staff and faculty ensure the student lounge facility in a traditional educational

setting, it is the responsibility of support staff and faculty to ensure the establishment and maintenance of the online social space environment. Faculty and staff are also responsible for the orientation of the student to the availability and use of the space. As participants of the community, the students are responsible for professional use of the established social space.

5. What are the "norms" of online learning?

5. Norms of online learning include stating standards/ground rules clearly in the course regarding expectations, e-mail messages, assignments, participation, discussions, due dates, evaluation, and grading system. Policies for clinical experience are also clearly described. Other norms are quality measures of online community including student support, faculty support, curriculum and instructions, and evaluation and assessment.

6. How do you promote etiquette in online community?

6. A welcome video and clearly posted instructions at the beginning of the term are initial steps to promote etiquette. Emphasis on reading materials posted before asking questions is also made. Informing students of office hours where e-mail messages might be sent and when reply could be expected is another step. Students are also advised to give their correct e-mail addresses to faculty and peers, and to update them if changes occur. In addition, they are encouraged to ask questions if they perceive that the written instructions are not clear.

7. How do you recognize and deal with anger?

7. Anger can be recognized from written comments, e-mail messages, or from other students. An e-mail message or a personal phone call to the involved student might help identify the reason for the anger. Communication that is not appropriate can also be managed by the group. Either the faculty or other participants can ask a general question such as "How is the conversation in this forum going?" or give "I" statements such as "I am uncomfortable about some of the conversation that is going on now in this forum" to elicit further identification of problems of group and individual communication. Dealing with angry or abusive remarks can become a way of modeling effective communication in online learning communities.

8. How do you handle comments that are offensive or biased?

8. Print a hard copy of the comments. Inform the involved student that his/her comments are not acceptable either through a phone call or an e-mail message. Be sure that online courses contain guidelines for handling offensive comments. Document those incidents.

9. How do you deal with students who are being disruptive in the online community?

9. Dealing with disruptive students is similar to dealing with students who write offensively. This includes adequate documentation, informing the involved student by a phone call or e-mail message that his/her behavior is unacceptable, and following the disciplinary guidelines that exist in the course, academic institution, or clinical agency.

10. What is socialization in an online community?

10. Socialization is a cornerstone of individuals living in a society. It involves being together, doing things together or sharing mutual interests. Socialization usually occurs by choice, although professionals socialize in work settings. Professional socialization is the process by which professional attitudes, values, and beliefs are developed to form the sense of identity and belonging to one's profession. In most schools of nursing, a program outcome about the development of professional values is included. Therefore, online learning needs to provide an opportunity for students to develop professionalism. Students in online courses can be socialized into a virtual community group. Students self-select professional and educational opportunities and bring groups together in an academic community. In the online community socialization is sharing information, experiences, goals, and dreams with colleagues.

11. Can you promote socialization in a distance environment?

11. Socialization can be promoted in online courses and programs. As students enter an online program, it is important to orient them to the similarities and differences of what to expect in the way of interpersonal relationships or social interactions. Interactions are very much a part of online learning. Formal interactions occur through posting of responses to assignments. This creates a professional socialization. Less formal interactions can take place through private e-mail or phone conversations.

Other types of socialization can be promoted in a distance environment, especially in nursing. Students have clinical experiences in all nursing programs that require an interface with agencies providing clinical opportunities. Agency staff or preceptors become partners and role models. Interpersonal relationships can become strong and help fill the gap, if any, of the face-to-face contact characterized as socialization.

Socialization in online courses also can be created by design by the use of group work and live chats. If students are required to work together, they reach out to others to build networks. Clinical assignments promote socialization through association with preceptors and other professional staff. Other types of assignments, such as interviews with clients or staff, promote socialization within the agency. Surveys can be used to assist learners identify their own values, and even to track the changes in their values and socialization throughout the course.

12. How do you write program/course/lesson objectives that deal with socialization to the profession for an online course?

12. Program outcomes related to communication encompass multiple aspects of socialization. Communication is a required outcome for accreditation of schools of nursing that must be extended beyond classroom settings. For example, "Uses communication skills in a variety of settings," is a broad program outcome that can be realized through online learning.

Course outcomes related to communication can reflect leveling of skills for writing, speaking, and evaluating professional social skills within programs. For example, a course outcome would state, "Evaluates communication skills in a professional setting." Socialization into the professional setting is an end product of effective communications.

A course unit objective that relates to a specific activity requiring interaction reflects socialization as a process. For example, an interview with an advanced practice nurse, regarding the integration of nursing research in practice, illustrates socialization into a practice role.

13. What teaching/learning activities promote socialization?

13. Any activity that requires interaction with a target population such as peers or colleagues promotes socialization. Assignments in online courses require weekly interactions among colleagues. Repeated interactions among people in the online community result in positive reinforcement, building socialization. Journals and reflection papers are other strategies. Due dates provide structure for keeping responses within a reasonable time frame.

14. How do you evaluate socialization in the online course?

14. Predetermined criteria for participation in course discussions, for example, length, depth, and quality, can be used to evaluate socialization. Educators can assign points to discussion postings and responses. Beyond the points, or requirements, the number and quality of voluntary responses in course discussions can be used to evaluate socialization. Positive, supportive entries support socialization and give the learner, peers, and educators a glimpse into the development of professional values as they are being developed. Journals and reflection papers as well as attitude/values clarification surveys are other evaluation strategies that work well when evaluating socialization. Another method of evaluating socialization or communication skills is through preceptor evaluation forms.

RESOURCES

Nesler, M. S., Hanner, M. B., Melburg, V., & McGowan, S. (2001). Professional socialization of baccalaureate nursing students: Can students in distance nursing programs be socialized? *Journal of Nursing Education, 40*(7), 293–302.

Miller, M. (2001). The effect of e-mail messages on student participation in the asynchronous online course. *Online Journal of Distance Learning Administration, 4*(3). Retrieved from: **www.westga.edu**

Section 8:
Teaching and E-Learning

Teaching in online communities is grounded in principles of good practice in education. Through active learning strategies, students conceptualize their own body of knowledge, test it, and apply it in clinical practice. The contributors to this unit introduce you to a variety of e-learning strategies and activities, and share their "tips" and tested strategies—ways to interact with learners, how to encourage learners to interact with each other, how to keep learning active, how to develop critical thinking abilities, and how to use online learning to support clinical teaching and learning. Learners in Web courses bring the same diversity to the online course as they do in the classroom. Effective e-teaching requires attention to inclusiveness and developing learners who are sensitive to others, effective communicators, aware of their own learning styles and needs, and culturally competent. Good teaching is good teaching regardless of the setting; in this unit you will learn how to take your expertise and experience from an onsite classroom to an online classroom.

Chapter 24: *Principles of Good Practice in E-Learning*

1. What are some guiding principles for good practice in an e-learning course?

1. Chickering and Gamson's (1987) seven principles of good practice in undergraduate education can be a concise way for educators to focus on the teaching and learning process as it occurs in an e learning environment. These principles, synthesized from educational research, are as follows:

1. Good practice encourages contacts between students and faculty.

2. Good practice develops reciprocity and cooperation among students.

3. Good practice uses active learning techniques.

4. Good practice gives prompt feedback.

5. Good practice emphasizes time on task.

6. Good practice communicates high expectations.

7. Good practice respects diverse talents and ways of learning.

2. Do I really need to take an active role in encouraging student contact with me in the e-learning environment?

2. One of the concerns in an e-learning environment is getting to know the student as an individual learner and as a member of the learning community. At the onset of the course, establish the expectations for communication and self-disclosure. Letting students know how often they can expect you to read their e-mail, when they can expect a response from you, how often they can expect feedback on their work, and how often they need to check the Web site for new information can go a long way toward keeping both you and the students satisfied with the communication process.

In a traditional class, students can have a look around and see who is in the class. If the technology is available, having one session early in the course where students can see one another in a real-time environment (for example, two-way video) can help learners meet and greet one another. If this is not available, faculty can have students share information about themselves as learners. By providing specific questions for students to answer, the faculty can help students focus their introductions to one another. This is a good first assignment for posting to the Web site. Attaching a photo can enhance the personalization of this communication.

3. *I find that I am inundated with e-mail from students. Help me get a perspective on this!*

3. One advantage of the asynchronous e-learning environment is that students can seek faculty at their convenience. There is no waiting for office hours, or cramming questions into the period just before or after a class session. Those students who have a more reflective and introspective personality in a typical classroom have an equal opportunity to be heard when taking an asynchronous e-learning class.

It is important to track the communication from students. In a face-to-face setting, the non-verbal cues can tell when a student is uninterested, confused, or out of touch with the learning activity. In the e-learning environment, the student who is not sending many messages could be having difficulty. It is the responsibility of the faculty member to be aware of the communication patterns from students and to look for cues that indicate a need for further support or encouragement. Don't forget that you can use the telephone! This real-time communication can go a long way to address problems or concerns that students have.

4. *How can I develop reciprocity and cooperation among the students in an e-learning course?*

4. The whole idea behind this principle is recognizing that there is a social aspect to learning. When assignments are designed for group work, it is important for the faculty to be sure the students have access to their cohort. If the course is administered via the Web, then students would meet in the virtual environment. If the course is offered at a distance location where the entire class meets, then the group activity should be geared to happen during assigned class time to avoid the complications inherent in the lives of distance students (many of whom are also working or have other responsibilities). Reporting back to the entire group the results of the problem-solving task is important for accountability, relevance, and ultimately validation for the learners. Whether through a verbal or written format, the process of explaining the solution causes students to discuss the analytic steps they took to solve the problem.

It is important for the faculty to be clear about the expectations and the evaluation process for group work. You will need to decide if the small groups can self-select or if you will arbitrarily assign students to the groups. You may even need to assign roles to various group members, depending on the experience of the learners. Be sure the time frames for the projects are clearly communicated.

5. *I keep hearing about active learning. Doesn't all learning require activity on the part of the learner?*

5. Technically, yes. But learning activities are not equal. When you hear educators talking about active learning, they usually are framing it in a cognitive constructivist viewpoint. In this paradigm the faculty becomes more of a guide for learning rather than the source of all knowledge. The learner is viewed as an active participant in the process.

For the faculty, emphasis is placed on knowing the learner and creating instruction so things will fall into place as the learner progresses through the instruction. Instruction is sequenced from the more concrete toward the more symbolic. Learners are encouraged to consider all the possibilities of the problem, to be creative, and to expand their analytical skills.

6. *How can I tell if I am using an active learning paradigm in my teaching?*

6. Look at your learning goals. They should require more than memorizing the information that you provided. Consider the ultimate goal of the curriculum. Will the learner be expected to use critical thinking? If so, build this into the course work.

Ask yourself these questions as you review learning activities:

- Is the learning situated in authentic tasks that are relevant to the students?

- Are students required to use cognitive skills to interpret experiences?

- Have you used any problem-based learning strategies such as case studies or simulations?

- Does the group work help learners negotiate the meaning of the concepts?

- Do learners report their findings back to larger class group?

- Do you use writing-to-learn strategies?

7. *I could spend hours giving feedback. What should I consider to keep my efforts in feedback focused?*

7. The first thing you should ask yourself is what is the purpose of feedback. The structure and timing of the feedback will depend on its purpose. Formative feedback would be the kind of feedback you give throughout the course to help students identify strengths, build confidence, and be challenged to reach the next level. Summative feedback is the evaluation of the end product of the course work and in most cases is the course grade.

Feedback may be for individuals or small groups. E-mail or phone conversations can work well for one-to-one feedback. E-mail works well to give group feedback. A considerable advantage to e-mail is the record it provides to both students and faculty as evidence of progress in the course. You may want to set up a computer-based tool to plan the frequency you will give detailed feedback to students, and to keep records of your feedback. In this way, you are sure to give feedback to each student on a regular basis, and it may prevent you from becoming overwhelmed at the large volume of student e-mail.

8. I don't understand what the principle about time on task is really about.

8. When you pay attention to time on task, you allocate realistic time for learning tasks and learners spend sufficient time to achieve learning outcomes. Faculty must recognize the energy and time required for learning to occur and be sure that assignments fit the course requirements. The realism that comes with constructivist learning experiences is countered by the constraints of time. It is important for the faculty to determine the ultimate goal of instruction. If the cognitive, intuitive, and inquiry skills are important goals, then the volume of content may be sacrificed. The value of deep knowledge of fewer content areas would be placed above a more superficial knowledge of more content areas.

9. How does time on task apply to the e-leaning environment?

9. An important consideration for e-learning is the technology you select for the task. Do students have the computer skills needed to be successful? If not, what accommodations have you made to see that they are ready?

Do not underestimate the learning curve, frustration, and failure factors. For example, if you want to use synchronous conferencing as a way to build group dynamics, you must determine if the site and server can manage the number of students you will have at any given time. You need to anticipate barriers for students who access from a remote site. Sometimes there is a maximum time for log-on to the system, or slow modem speeds that may preclude their timely input to a discussion. Is there a dial-up number that students can use if they have computer glitches during a synchronous chat time? You will want to cultivate a strong working relationship with the computer support person and give this person a "heads up" when you plan synchronous activities.

Another application of this principle is considering the focus of assignments and removing unnecessary barriers for the students. For example, a faculty member who asks students to critique various Internet resources would set up a Web page with hot links to decrease student time in accessing the resources.

10. How can I set high expectations in a Web course?

10. Clearly communicate the expectations at the onset. One way to do this is to discuss what you expect for A level work, B level work, and so on, and clearly describe what is considered unsatisfactory work. Another more positive way to state this is to use the statement "An outstanding student will…" You might provide several examples of work that varies in quality for students to critique to help them understand the grading criteria.

Use the feedback process to stimulate students to move to the next level and to help them recognize for themselves their progress during the course. It is always important to frame assignments in such a way that students can see the relevance of the assignment to their professional growth.

I believe in frequent feedback—both positive and constructive—early in the course. I also ask students to self-evaluate. This helps them to internalize the performance criteria—and builds a professional skill. Peer review is another strategy for enhancing high expectations. When students know their work is to be made public, they may strive to make it their best work.

11. How can I tailor an e-learning course to accommodate the diverse talents and learning styles of students?

11. First of all, you need to increase students' self-awareness of their learning styles and strengths. This may include formal or informal methods. Some schools have students complete a Myers-Briggs inventory as they enter the program. This information is useful for both faculty and students in understanding how they approach the course. Using a formal learning inventory is another option. Students can be asked to self-assess for both successful learning strategies as well as their perceived barriers to learning. However it is obtained, this information is helpful for both faculty and students as they progress through the course.

When faculty use a variety of strategies for learning, students are more likely to encounter a strategy that is successful. In the same way, faculty should use multiple measures and sources for evaluation of students. Thus, students are not penalized if they are weaker in one of the methods of learning or evaluation. Evaluation and feedback are useful as they help students recognize progress in learning throughout the course.

RESOURCES

Bonk, C. J., & King, K. S. (Eds.). (1998). *Electronic collaborators*. Mahwah, NJ: Lawrence Erlbaum Associates.

Chickering, A. W., & Ehrmann, S. (1996*). Implementing the seven principles: Technology as lever*. Retrieved from **http://www.tltgroup.org/ehrmann.htm**

Chickering, A. W., & Gamson, Z. F. (1987). Seven principles for good practice in undergraduate education. *AAHE Bulletin, 39*(7), 3–6.

Erhmann, S. (1995). Asking the right questions: What does research tell us about technology and higher learning? *Change, 27*(2), 20–27.

Novotny, J. (Ed.). (1999). *Distance learning in nursing*. New York: Springer Publishing.

Whitis, G. (2001). *A survey of technology-based distance education: Emerging issues and lessons learned*. Washington, DC: Association of Academic Health Centers.

Chapter 25: *E-Learning Activities and Adventures*

1. What do you mean by e-learning activities and adventures?

1. The primary prompt for learning in Web courses is thoughtfully constructed learning activities. Because of the nature of the online learning community, it is possible to incorporate learning activities that include group work, links, use of multimedia, and interaction and are, in fact, so much fun, that they become "adventures."

2. What encourages the students to engage in e-learning activities and give their best efforts?

2. Students become engaged when you place assignments in the discussion forums. Students can see each others' work and discuss differences. They respond to feedback and encouragement—send them a group or private e-mail to let them know they are meeting course goals.

3. What types of e-learning activities increase student-to-student interaction?

3. Encourage online study groups with division of labor for solving case studies, answering questions, or preparing for exams; have students e-mail each other their work or post it to the discussion forum or shared workspace. Choose activities that can be done in small groups. When you use small groups, consider the pros and cons of assigning groups ahead of time; rotate group members for various activities. Be sure to weigh the advantages of group work and allow sufficient course time to work in groups to complete the assignment. Debates, case studies, simulations, and problem-solving activities are easily (and best) done in groups and provide students an opportunity to interact. Ask thought provoking and controversial questions that stimulate lively interaction and elicit a variety of opinions.

4. How do you stimulate curiosity to pursue a topic further?

4. Not every student has enormous interest in every topic, but on the other hand there will usually be several students who want more information about a topic, or realize they need to learn about the topic from another angle. Having meaningful optional learning experiences available makes good use of Web-based learning. You can provide links to interesting Web pages to facilitate exploration, or you can suggest additional readings. You can also create activities that take the learner into the clinical practice arena to have a dialogue with a patient or a nurse to learn more about the topic.

5. How can you design learning activities to accommodate differences in learning styles?

5. Students learn in various ways, and it will be important for you to design learning activities that respect this diversity. For visual style learners, you could incorporate videos for difficult topics, such as pathophysiology or selected skills. Many Web sites have video clips to which

you can link. For auditory style learners, you could use narrated PowerPoint slides or audio clips. You can also encourage telephone interaction or study groups in which students explain material to each other. For learners who require direction and concrete examples, design the learning activities to include these. Some students prefer to have the teacher or expert available to validate their work; Web courses are ideal for these learners as someone, either the teacher or a classmate with an answer, is only an e-mail away.

6. How do you introduce variety into learning activities?

6. Using the same type of learning experiences for each lesson becomes boring quickly! Incorporate crossword puzzles and matching games into course activities. Search published test bank materials for games, or use software designed to generate online puzzles. Alternate individual activities with pairs or small groups. Ask students to develop or suggest learning activities for the course. Invite a guest expert to join the class for a session.

7. How do you plan activities for different domains of learning?

7. For the affective domain, have students share their own values in relation to topics such as disease prevention and perceived personal barriers to health promotion. Encourage learners to share their responses online.

For the cognitive domain, have students work in groups to answer patient care case study guided questions. Practice tests also facilitate cognitive domain learning as the learner can practice and obtain immediate feedback which can be provided in most online testing software.

For the psychomotor domain, tap into interactive software and virtual reality (such as placing leads for an ECG). You may wish to require learners to purchase or have access to these skills demonstrations on CD-ROM; and some skills demonstrations may be available on various Web sites and you can link to those.

8. What helps students with a sense of control in the class?

8. Students need to experience a sense of control and ability to give input to the direction of the course. Be sure to provide this same opportunity in a Web course. For example, when there is a request for a change in a test date, use an online survey or hold a discussion in a separate forum to allow everyone to participate in the decision, whether present at that particular time or not.

9. *How can you help students evaluate the effectiveness of their study techniques?*

9. Learning activities are designed to assist students to accomplish course goals and achieve course competencies, but in Web courses, students have difficulty being certain they are studying the "right way" or the "right thing." Giving students feedback about how well they are completing learning activities is essential. You can report to students their percentage achievement on each class topic. Load this in an online grade book that the student can print individually. Report their percentage achievement on each course competency across the different units in the course and load this in an online grade book as well. In individual exam review, note unit topics that are well achieved versus less well achieved. Help the student apply techniques from well achieved units to other areas. Note strengths and weaknesses in achievement of course competencies and point out strong areas to support student confidence and encourage transfer of techniques to other course competencies.

10. *How can you encourage students to study for exams?*

10. Testing must be linked to the course objectives or competencies and the learning activities. Again, because Web courses can be isolating, you can give learners "tips" about how to prepare for the exam. For example, you can provide test maps, with review questions online for each exam item. A test map usually points to the content item and course competency addressed by each test item. Encourage students to use the test map file to enter their own answers to the test map review questions and submit for feedback.

11. *How can you determine the student's grasp of material?*

11. Give rapid feedback on test map review question answers. Correct inaccuracies and encourage increased depth in responses as needed. Help students learn to recognize when they do and do not grasp the material. Students can also give feedback to each other; you can encourage students to form study groups so they can give feedback to each other.

12. *How can you help with test anxiety?*

12. Provide an online discussion forum the night before exams; announce specific times faculty will be in the forum to respond to questions about the exam. Indicate e-mail is available for questions as well if students do not want their question aired in the open discussion forum.

13. *What activities help with test-taking skills?*

13. Provide practice exams in online format that provide feedback for correct answers including an explanation of the rationale. Set the exam for multiple attempts by students. You can also include in feedback an explanation of why incorrect responses are incorrect.

RESOURCE

Cartwright, J. (2000). Lessons learned: Using asynchronous computer-mediated conferencing to facilitate group discussion. *Journal of Nursing Education, 39*(2), 87–90.

Chapter 26: *Critical Thinking*

1. *What is critical thinking?*

1. Critical thinking (CT) is a complex process of learning. Individuals incorporate various aspects of learning involving not only cognitive abilities but also attitudes and skills. Learners can be reflective and further develop a method of inquiry that promotes learning beyond professional roles using analysis, synthesis, evaluation, and inference. It is critical for individuals to discriminate between facts and beliefs and, ultimately, come to their own conclusions. Critical thinking enhances the process of questioning the meaning of observations against standards of practice. E-learners are guided to seek alternative methods for problem solving. As a result, learners become more competent, insightful, and reflective professionals.

   E-learning can strengthen the exploration of situations and problems and assist in the discovery of options. Opportunities for developing skills with situations (e.g., case studies, computer simulations, and discussion forums) assist with the process of selecting relevant clinical information, inferring potential problems, and taking appropriate action.

2. *How can you develop critical thinking skills in an online learning community?*

2. The process of learning to develop critical thinking begins with guiding the learner to become familiar with (1) the resources available for online learning, (2) continuing education courses, (3) online opportunities for communicating with other health professionals (e.g., electronic bulletin boards), and (4) online resources that supplement learning and have clinical applications. Online novices often need guidance and support to acquire skills appropriate for online discussions. Whether they participate solely for professional development or personal fulfillment, learners may need assistance in using online tools. The nurse educator also assumes a new role in modeling critical thinking behaviors and developing student-directed activities that promote learning.

3. *Why are critical thinking strategies important in creating a productive online learning experience?*

3. CT strategies enhance the learner's interest and the anticipation that is created by stimulating critical thinking and further peak the learner's interest for subsequent learning. Critical thinking activities involve active learning, thus creating better retention of content. From the educator's perspective, critical thinking activities can be helpful in assessing competence versus

incompetence. Ultimately, learners enjoying the online activity will want to participate in similar types of experiences.

4. What is the educator's role in promoting CT in an online learning community?

4. The challenge for the educator is in facilitating and promoting the online learning experience. The educator's role is one of developer, designer, and director of the learning process. Initially, the goals and outcomes for an online learning experience must be developed. In order to promote the individual's comfort level with e-learning strategies, educators need to pre-assess the learner. The format then proceeds from design to implementation, management, and evaluation of the technology appropriate for learning.

The educator's role is continued throughout the learning activity with guided learning questions and discussions to promote analysis and discovery. The success of the e-learning experience is enhanced through the teacher's role as coach and collaborator.

5. What are examples of online activities that promote CT?

5. A variety of online learning activities can be adapted from traditional learning formats. The use of case studies with prompted student responses lends itself well to this format, especially if a group of learners is participating in the same case analysis. Creating online scenarios that offer alternate solutions challenges learners toward more effective problem solving. This can be accomplished by asking learners what they believe the problem is and what data support the problem solving.

Traditional teaching methods offer limited learner engagement. However, having access to materials from wide varieties of Web resources demonstrates a new modality of gaining the most up-to-date information across continents. Educators can pose scenarios asking each Web participant to play various roles of a case study and present ideas from that role's perspective. The possibilities for teaching/learning activities online are limitless.

6. How can synchronous online discussion formats facilitate critical thinking?

6. Synchronous and asynchronous discussions differ in that they occur in different online time frames. Synchronous refers to a "real time" mode, where all participants are online at the same time. This format is similar to chat rooms or discussion boards occurring with all participants online together forming a group. Ideas can be brainstormed and further stimulate others' modes of

thinking. Supplemental classroom activities, such as synchronous chat rooms, allow frequent opportunities for learners to further explore ideas and support consensus and decision making.

7. *How can asynchronous online discussion formats facilitate critical thinking?*

7. The asynchronous format allows learners to work at their own pace and at any time. The participants find it advantageous to have adequate time to process their thoughts and respond to others or the online query without having to give an immediate response. Many introspective learners appreciate this format. Some e-learners can feel intimidated by face-to-face discussion, while they may find it easier to challenge others' thoughts and ideas in an online environment. Asynchronous online discussion is ideal for small groups of persons to interact effectively.

8. *What are peer-participant critiques?*

8. Peer-participant critiques are guided learning experiences that promote and encourage personal analysis of situations, cooperative learning, and reflective thinking. Learners' growth is enhanced when peers provide constructive feedback and promote discussion that builds on each other's comments. Ultimately, participants see others' points of view and work collaboratively toward improved decision making.

9. *How do you organize peer-participant critiques as an online learning community?*

9. In an online learning community there are choices available to the learner that can be individualized or applied to online groups. Individually, the learner can strengthen personal skills in an area of practice and apply those skills to past and future learning. A group online discussion promotes critical thinking and offers opportunities to share experiences and personal views, and facilitates feedback to others in the e-learning community. However, limiting group size provides for a more productive online interaction. Well-developed interactive learning activities decrease the learner's perception of isolation and create a sense of community among learners.

10. *What are the advantages of online activities in promoting peer-participant critiques?*

10. Advantages to electronic communication are that it is instantaneous and it promotes immediate learning. Online activities encourage communication with peers. Through peer interactions, there are opportunities to consider various options and brainstorm actions and consequences of a situation.

11. *Are there any disadvantages to using peer-participant critiques in the online learning community?*

11. There are also disadvantages to e-learning. In working alone, the learner is not interrelating with others. Another disadvantage is that facial expressions and other non-verbal cues are lacking. Consequently, these participants lack traditional communication feedback techniques.

12. *How does critical thinking increase problem solving in clinical practice?*

12. Novice nurses need opportunities to dialogue with experienced nurses acting as mentors. Clinical decision making is developed over time; problem solving requires a balance of clinical reasoning and practiced judgments. Staff nurses challenged with complex clinical situations may consult online experts and refer to online library resources. Improved access of readily available materials allows clinicians to remain current in their practice. Furthermore, educators can design computer-based activities to dialogue productively with staff and share their expertise with others.

13. *How do you evaluate CT?*

13. Traditional methods used for both objective and subjective evaluations can also be accomplished in an electronic environment. Technology presents limitations for test security if the learner takes the exams online in a non-proctored setting and the course grade is highly dependent on evaluating actual learning. However, the basis for both formative and summative evaluations is multi-faceted. In adult learning theory, online educators act primarily as facilitators, while the individual's participation is promoted largely by using criteria that match the learners' needs and address clear learning outcomes. Online assessment rubrics can be established to address three major areas: (1) content, (2) expression of ideas, and (3) participation online. Within each area, Likert-scales subcategorize expected behaviors for each concept, and include a critical thinking component as part of each rubric. Learners anticipating the expectation of incorporating critical thinking will likely strive to meet that standard.

14. *How can critical thinking promote global healthcare issues and influence the future of nursing through e-learning?*

14. Complex healthcare challenges require nurses to be skilled at thinking critically. Global healthcare issues require solutions that incorporate worldwide nursing perspectives. Situations can be presented online, inviting cross-disciplinary input, for in-depth analyses. Nurses from all specialties and across the generations can collaborate electronically on issues that affect the health of the world. Prior to the 20th century, countries have had a tunnel-vision approach to world healthcare issues. Given the future of health care and its many challenges, no nurse or group of nurses can afford to be so ethnocentric. While developing nations may have had the economic resources to research health care more thoroughly, underdeveloped nations have a cohort of nurses who deeply understand the culture and the factors that promote or impede collective problem solving. The online environment can decrease the geographic challenges and open a forum for constructive problem solving, worldwide.

15. Are there limits to using e-learning activities to develop critical thinking?

15. Limitations to using e-learning include the following:

- Individuals must have access to the technology and be able to understand the purpose of the e-learning activity. Electronic transmission problems and lack of computer support can pose major obstacles.

- The learner's positive attitude toward e-learning is essential. Users who have near phobias about computers need extra guidance and support to initially increase their comfort levels with this format.

- Some students or learners may have a difficult time with self-disclosure via e-learning.

- When using e-learning, confidentiality of discussions is difficult to maintain.

- Organizing and updating e-learning activities and providing feedback to learners is labor intensive. Additionally, there might be a need for educational consultants.

- The e-learning activity designers may need release time or financial compensation for their expertise.

16. What e-learning strategies can the educator use to promote the learner's growth through reflective-learning activities?

16. Guided learning and use of case studies can promote reflective learning. Allowing the learners time to review online discussions can increase professional competence, self-confidence, and reflective clinical practice. Learners need to develop such skills with ongoing self-assessment.

17. With the lack of traditional verbal cueing, how can e-learning promote critical thinking?

17. Principles of open communication pertain to online discussions. Being in tune with others' online comments and responding to questions or concerns that have been raised offer validation that the question is of interest to the learner. If comments or questions seem confusing to the group or might be interpreted differently, this should be addressed. Participants closing their own comments with a question, such as "How do the rest of you feel?" promote further conversation for discussion and critique. If the assignment is a graded activity, educators might build in course credit for dissenting ideas or thought-provoking discussions. Traditional typewritten characters are widely familiar to most e-mail users and substitute in electronic formats as common facial and nonverbal cues (e.g., an electronic symbol **:-)** acts as a smile).

RESOURCES

Bartels, J. E. (1998). Developing reflective learners—student self-assessment as learning. *Journal of Professional Nursing, 14*(3), 135.

Chubinski, S. (1996). Creative critical-thinking strategies. *Nurse Educator, 21*(6), 23–27.

Cunningham, H., & Plotkin, K. (2000). Using the Internet in a nursing clinical practicum course: Benefits and challenges. *The Australian Electronic Journal of Nursing Education, 5*(2), 1–8.

Glendon, K., & Ulrich, D. I. (1997). Unfolding cases: An experienced learning model. *Nurse Educator, 22*(4), 15–18.

Green, C. (2000). *Critical thinking in nursing.* New Jersey: Prentice-Hall, Inc.

Malloy, S. E , & DeNatale, M. L. (2001). Online critical thinking: A case study analysis. *Nurse Educator, 26*(4), 191–197.

Pesut, D., & Herman, J. (1999). *Clinical reasoning: The art and science of critical and creative thinking.* New York: Delmar Publishers.

Weiss, R. E., Knowlton, D. S., & Speck, B. W. (2000). *Principles of effective teaching in the online classroom.* San Francisco: Jossey-Bass.

Weis, P. A., & Guyton-Simmons, J. A. (1998). Computer simulation for teaching critical-thinking skills. *Nurse Educator, 23*(2), 30–33.

Chapter 27: *E-Learning and the Clinical Practicum*

1. How can I use e-learning to facilitate clinical learning experiences?

1. Although educators may not think that Web course tools are used in clinical teaching, learning, and evaluation, they can, in fact, be very useful. For example, these tools can be used to help students prepare for clinical experience, to communicate with the clinical agency, to access learning resources, to access clinical agency information, and to evaluate the outcomes of the experience.

2. What information can I communicate electronically to clinical sites as preparation for student experiences?

2. Copies of syllabi, evaluation tools, clinical schedules, announcements that affect the clinical units, and any last minute updates are easily transmitted via e-mail. Student performance expectations and guidelines for staff nurses when working with students are additional materials that can be sent by e-mail to individual staff members or to the unit in general. For sites that use preceptors or where there is less faculty/staff interaction, e-mail is particularly useful. Information is rapidly transmitted by e-mail and a record of the transfer of information is available should the need arise.

3. What do I need to think about when talking about student access and use of computer systems?

3. Five years ago, the question to students was, "Do you have access to computers?" This has evolved into how sophisticated is the technology used by students and faculty. As clinical faculty, be clear about what students have access to and can use readily before they need to use it in a clinical course. Students often become frustrated and dissatisfied with technology so continued learning about technology is imperative. Once established, technology support for students and faculty helps with resolving problems.

4. How can e-learning help with client research prior to clinical experience?

4. Faculty can use e-mail to transmit student assignments for the next clinical day. This is particularly useful for students who are geographically isolated. Care must be taken to ensure patient confidentiality by deleting any identifying information before transmission.

A follow-up e-learning strategy is a synchronous preconference discussion for students before clinical experiences. Ideally it is student-led in a collaborative learning environment with faculty serving as coach and resource. This is a great way to see plans of care and student timelines. It is an excellent means to view the thinking of students as they prepare for clinical experiences so there are few surprises on the morning of the clinical experience.

5. What are some of the electronic resources available to students in clinical agencies?

5. Resources in hospital systems vary and students' access to computer services in most agencies is limited and available only through faculty or staff. Here is a list of what may be accessible at an institution:

- Policy and procedure manuals online and readily accessible to employees.

- Drug/medication guides for staff, much like a drug manual.

- Patient education materials created or purchased by the institution. Using standardized materials provides diagnosis, institution and physician consistency, and assumes hospital approval. However, these must be individualized to each client.

- Purchased multidisciplinary care management systems in standardized languages (e.g., care plans and pathways).

- Round reports, Kardex, labs, physician orders, medical diagnosis profiles.

- Telephone translation services are particularly useful in multicultural settings.

- Computerized documentation of client care is becoming more widespread. It will be essential that students become familiar with this type of documentation.

6. How can students find the most current information and materials electronically in preparation for or during clinical experiences?

6. Students can find information through:

- Searches on their home computer with Web access

- Electronic updates to complement textbooks

- Professional Web searches through library systems

- Searches of national databases by profession and area of focus or through the federal government

- Online journals with full texts or abstracts available

- CD-ROM or computer disks available with texts

- Nursing care plans and care pathways on the Web

7. How can students review previously acquired information and skills electronically?

7. There are synchronous or asynchronous professional forums, continuing education offerings, video conferencing online, professional videotapes in hospitals, and programming for patients, students, and staff. All are means to share information.

Many schools use:

- IAVDs (Interactive video discs) that place students in a clinical situation and ask them to assess, diagnose, plan, implement, and evaluate care

- CD-ROMs to teach and assess psychomotor skills

- Most disciplines in nursing and organizations associated with nursing have Web sites. Simply identifying the skill on a Web search will identify many of those sites and then it is up to the students to determine what is best for them. Another great starting point is faculties who often have lists of Web sites that are excellent student resources.

8. What are other e-learning strategies to promote clinical competency?

8.
- Use electronic case studies developed by students or instructors or from Web sources that can be unfolding or presented at one time.

- Bring in specialists who may not be available to meet with students face-to-face but are willing to enter asynchronous discussions to teach, provide clarity, or stimulate discussion (e.g., clinical nurse specialists, physicians, social workers).

- Consider clinical electronic journaling: Reflection on practice helps students transfer information from the ideal of theory to the practicality of clinical exposure. The electronic format provides privacy for honest discussion with faculty. Faculty can use generic questions to stimulate thinking: What experience helped you to grow/learn most this week? How will you prepare differently for your next clinical experience? Sequence the journals so students can reflect and view the changes as they progress through the semester.

- Use students as resources for one another in a discussion forum. This interactive process reinforces the teaching/learning process, reflection, and affective domain development.

9. How do you conduct "post conferences" online?

9. Different types of post conferences can be handled electronically but establish ground rules first. Determine a time line (for everyone's sanity) and an agenda. Students are often tired after clinical experiences, so planning the conference in the evening after family concerns are taken care of works well.

This also offers time to reflect before the discussion.

Types of post conferences:

a. **Clinical group post conference.** A synchronous discussion (chat room) relevant to the day's events. Faculty and students can see flow of thought, identify accuracy or errors in thinking, and summarize the clinical day right before their eyes.

b. **One-on-one conference about assignments.** After grading student papers, an electronic discussion about the paper is helpful especially if there is a long time before you will see the student in person.

c. **"Intermediate" e-learning conference for back-to-back clinical experiences.** An e-learning conference scheduled as a chat room or discussion forum with all students is especially useful after the first day of clinicals if there are two clinical days back to back. Identification of need for changes in the following clinical experience, addressing recognized weaknesses in student understanding of clinical issues, patient care or diagnoses, clarification of issues affecting all students, or a well-deserved pat on the back are all possible electronically.

d. **Issue conferences.** Asynchronous conferencing focused on a student or faculty identified issue. As the rotation progresses, all other students contribute to the discussion. This promotes listening to peers and critical thinking by all students about an issue only one student may have experience with. This collective learning is broader than individual effort. Conference guidelines including time and content need to be set by the instructor so that everything is very clear to the student. Particularly important are the timelines. Students often wait until the last minute to join this forum, misunderstand what needs to be done, and do not read each other's contributions.

10. How do students conduct a peer critique online?

10. Any paperwork submitted electronically to faculty could be peer reviewed technically. I provide students with electronic access to all official forms used in the clinical experience. The completed forms can be sent as attachments to students as well as faculty. Reviewers can use a different color ink to identify their input. This review can be substituted for a post conference or paper but

adequate time for student contemplation and response is needed.

Peer critique can be used with care plans, pathways, and assessments. Asking for evidence-based information to validate comments makes it a more studious process. The faculty member will monitor the online discussion for quality and participation. If a respondent is not contributing adequately, contact the individual to inform him/her to increase the number and quality of comments. Students tend to avoid being critical of one another; this is always a disadvantage of the peer review process.

11. How does a learner develop and maintain a record of clinical experiences?

11. Learners can record their achievements in one course or develop a portfolio of their clinical accomplishments to take into practice. At the beginning of each course, the student is provided with an electronic format or skeleton to record clinical experience, which would include:

1. Psychomotor skills (list with level of skill performance)

2. Lists of clients, age, diagnoses, nursing focus, and so on

3. Examples of electronically submitted papers for the course (e.g., care pathways)

This can be used by the student for self-assessment of needed clinical experiences at the beginning, middle, and end of each course and semester to reflect progression through the curriculum. This encourages analysis, planning for improvement, and self-evaluation of learning and provides evidence of practicum competency. The clinical instructor or preceptor can review progress with the learner for verification and offer suggestions for further development at any time during the courses. Students should be held responsible for maintaining this record of clinical experiences. Electronic portfolios for each student require much larger computer storage space and usually are a cooperative effort between student and school of nursing.

12. How can I give the learner feedback about clinical experiences?

12. The educator should provide feedback to the student by computer shortly after experiences are completed. It is wise to use the official clinical evaluation tool so the student can see expected performance and where the student is as compared to what is expected. The student can reflect on his/her achievement of these competencies. Because the educator can give this feedback to the student in rapid turnaround time, the student can react, reflect, and plan responses for experiences that follow. This also becomes the written record of critical incidents. The privacy of this forum allows the student to receive feedback on clinical performance with an added sense of safety. Even if more consultation is needed, the face-to-face conference time is streamlined.

Self-journaling by the student is a more personal and emotional record of clinical experiences. The educator's comments to a journal can help validate or refute a student's reflection, give a more realistic perspective to the student's self-evaluation of performance, and help direct more realistic plans for improvement.

13. How do I evaluate students clinically online?

13. The same formats used in person-to-person conferences can be used online. The formative and summative computerized evaluation of a student's performance, if done electronically each week throughout the clinical experiences, offers no surprises to the student. Students appreciate evaluation of performance online as it is timely and always accessible. Initially, the student has access to the blank evaluation form containing the expected competencies for the course. By the end of the course, the student sees the incremental feedback/evaluations and then a summary of his/her progress to meet competencies. Again, these formats allow the student to read, reflect, identify concerns, and develop a plan based on identified strengths and weaknesses. When the student and instructor meet face-to-face, both are ready for a focused conference that addresses present problems, strategies for change, and future directions.

14. Are there any problems with online clinical evaluations?

14. Computerized student evaluations carry hazards. Since the instructor is not present to interpret the evaluation verbally, the student may misunderstand or incorrectly interpret comments on the evaluation. Electronically, the faculty is not there to diffuse or reinterpret these situations. This creates the need for a person-to-person conference, which will require more time later. Learning contracts or agreements are examples of this. Any evaluation or learning situation that potentially exposes emotions or creates vulnerability for the student must be handled in a face-to-face conference. Initial communication with students about negative situations can occur online though. This documents that notification has occurred and provides a written record. Copies of evaluations and incidents can be stored in a central location (LAN) and can be available to the student and faculty for future reference.

15. What other information is available to supplement faculty evaluation of students?

15. Compliments or concerns about a student's performance or interactions can be sent to the instructor by e-mail from staff nurses and preceptors. Such communication MUST be kept private and anonymous in order to maintain objectivity. These communications may not contain specific data but can motivate the instructor to contact the student for a face-to-face exchange of information. If you are soliciting information from staff about student performance, do let students know in advance.

As an alternative, the instructor can invite staff comments by sending a list of questions or requesting input from persons who worked with students during a clinical rotation. This process can be formalized or can remain relatively casual.

16. How can students do online evaluations of the clinical course, faculty, clinical experiences, and preceptors?

16. Anonymous course and instructor evaluations can be made available for a limited and specific period of time to students to complete online. Quantitative results can be combined from the provided rating scale and presented as a numerical point, or percentage, on that scale. Qualitative comments can be listed electronically without identifying the student. These compiled results can then be reviewed online by faculty and/or administrators. Students really like the anonymity as well as the convenience of being able to complete evaluations when it is convenient for them.

17. Are there any disadvantages to online faculty, course, or agency evaluations?

17. Students may choose not to take the time to complete an online evaluation since they do it on their own time. It is difficult to hold students accountable for completion of the evaluation because of the anonymity and inability to track responders. Also students may fear the evaluations are not anonymous despite instructor assurances.

18. How can the computer be used for hospital and agency record keeping and evaluation?

18. Online use of education/training record keeping for hospital and agency staff can also occur as described for students. These data can be useful to staff development educators, inservice presenters, and managers for improving and monitoring the quality of educational offerings and record keeping.

Online evaluation of training and educational experiences can be completed with the same anonymity as seen with faculty or course evaluations in the collegiate setting. Evaluation of orientation sessions, mandatory inservice programs/education, practice updates, and certifications (e.g., CPR) can all be facilitated electronically. Another effective use for hospitals and agencies is to create and maintain staff records online, benefiting the individual employee as well as nursing management. Each staff member has a computerized record of training, certifications, continuing education attendance, positive and negative incidences, and self/administrative evaluation. These e-files will be clear and succinct in providing evidence for evaluation and assist in planning individual direction for career goals and institutional reward.

The databases can be linked. With this in place, when an attendance list for an inservice program is entered into the database, it is reflected in the employee's file.

19. Are there any instances where clinical information is not meant for an online format?

19. Issues involving strong emotions where non-verbal contact and ability to monitor responses are essential, such as death and abuse, are not appropriate online. Discussion about poor performance or unsafe practice should not be done online. All computer communication must be considered retrievable and reviewable by anyone; therefore, privacy becomes a critical concern.

20. What are the legal implications of using the computer for clinical experiences?

20. All persons communicating by computer must maintain confidentiality and privacy of patient information. Working in a secured, password protected, or encrypted environment protects confidentiality. Other privacy issues everyone needs to be concerned with include sharing passwords, sitting at the computer with friends who may share information, and use of voice software. Computers in public spaces such as libraries allow information to be more accessible to bystanders.

Copyright of Web sources and computer accessible material must be observed by students as well as faculty. All must know how to work with public domain materials and credit sources correctly.

There is often the temptation for inappropriate use of computer time, paper, and other resources available online. Playing games on the computer, plagiarism, writing papers for another individual, and use of inappropriate material are all examples. The instructor must be aware of potential concerns and prepare the students to be responsible and accountable for their computer actions.

RESOURCES

Elfrink, V. L., Davis, L. S., Fitzwater, E., Castleman, J., Burley, J., Gorney-Moreno, M. J., et al. (2000). A comparison of teaching strategies for integrating information technology into clinical nursing education. *Nurse Educator, 25*(3), 136–144.

DeBourgh, G. A. (2001). Using Web technology in a clinical nursing course. *Nurse Educator, 26,* 227–233.

DeNatale, M. L., & Malloy, S. (2001). Online critical thinking: A case study analysis. *Nurse Educator, 26*(4), 191–197.

Kennerly, S. (2001). Fostering interaction through multimedia. *Nurse Educator, 26*(4), 90–94.

Chapter 28: *Inclusive Teaching Online*

1. *What is inclusive teaching?*

1. Inclusive teaching emphasizes helping students learn by using multiple perspectives and multiple instructional strategies, thus helping students learn more about themselves as unique individuals and as members of a diverse community. The terms "culturally relevant," "multicultural education," and "teaching diversity" are broad synonyms for appealing to diverse learners with a variety of approaches.

2. *Where do I start?*

2. Identify what areas of diversity are easy and uneasy for you. If you are comfortable with variation in learning styles or basic principles for dealing with cultural diversity, build your repertoire. Conduct a self-assessment and a class evaluation on your own use of multiple activities, cultural content, and your relationship to students from all backgrounds. You should also begin to decide what culturally-based skills and attitudes students should be able to apply to the courses and clinical experiences. This list may include the flexible use of terminology, display of empathy in assignments, active listening, and critical thinking about ideas and people involved.

3. *How do I establish a climate of respect for diversity in an online course?*

3. Begin with a statement of optimism like, "Difference can separate. But we are going to use it to build our online community." Share your cultural experiences such as travel, research, or personal observations that have informed your knowledge of cultural differences. Invite students to become co-researchers on departmental, community-based projects. Let students know that you are committed to learning more about your own values, assumptions, and biases. Post or ask students to post quotes on difference, community, and similarity throughout the semester.

4. *How do I motivate learners to appreciate cultural differences?*

4. Ask students what they want to learn about cultural diversity. If they admit no gaps in their knowledge base, give them scenarios or simulations where they have to consider cultural competence. Ask them to post a list of a homogeneous and a heterogeneous group. Ask them to explore the possible differences and similarities that they may find in both. Use any activities where learners explore their definition and notions of difference. Also, rely on professional sites that display experts speaking out about the importance of cultural awareness and cultural sensitivity in the health professions and Web

5. **How can I get learners to increase their awareness of their social identity?**

5. Ask students to introduce themselves integrating at least four different significant roles. Use activities that ask them to offer experiences where their roles were perceived positively and negatively. You could also have students fill in their perception of safe and unsafe zones for dialogues on identity and society (see Figure 1). After they identify the broad issues that each zone includes, have students brainstorm possible intrapersonal strategies for moving an unsafe topic to the safe zone.

Figure 1. **Diversity Zone Activity**

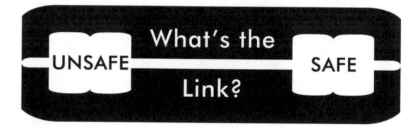

6. **How can I get learners to increase their own awareness about how they relate to others?**

6. After learners discuss personal strategies for dealing with "unsafe" topics, discuss ways to integrate cultural awareness into their professional development plan. Also, consistently ask for feedback on their comfort level with multiple perspectives and the lessons they learned from interaction with other students and with nurses in clinical practice.

7. **How can I encourage learners to reveal insights about themselves and others?**

7. Emphasize self-knowledge in the form of learning styles, family values, and personality traits as it affects individual and group work. Probe students' past experiences as a way for them to assess whether or not the course offers new and useful information and whether or not they have learned. Also, allow students to process group work in the areas of negotiation and sensitivity to difference.

8. **Shall I require learners to provide information about their cultural background?**

8. No, if students feel like they are being forced to reveal their social and cultural identities, both students and the classroom dynamic will suffer. Students should never feel that the amount of disclosure affects their final grade in the course. The critical aspect of cultural competence

sites that present voices of patients and clients who have constructive comments for healthcare workers.

is to know one's own social identity, to be able to reflect upon interactions with others, and revise certain notions that hinder cross-cultural communication. Require some interaction with unfamiliar territory and feedback on the process. Also, require understanding of certain principles and integration of cultural competence in class assignments.

9. How do I initiate a discussion about a sensitive topic?

9. Survey students' comfort level with social and cultural identities. Allow students to e-mail you early (and throughout the course, if needed) to discuss their ideas before they present them to the class. Ask students to post a one-sentence opinion, definition, or question about the topic. Post a link to a news clipping that may provoke some immediate reactions. Ask students to respond to the sensitive topic presented. Also, use short video clips to demonstrate diverse narratives and cases. If students meet in class, get permission to videotape a discussion for future classes or for their own end-of-the-semester reflection.

10. How do I de-escalate conflict in a discussion forum?

10. Reinforce student-and-teacher generated rules for engagement. Encourage students to reinforce them as well. Deal immediately with subtle and overt comments that are perceived negatively. Allow students to complete their thoughts. Make sure you clarify their ideas by paraphrasing them. If students are being isolated or becoming the focus of negative feedback, acknowledge the frustration of discussing issues of difference. However, give students an opportunity to research these ideas rather than focus solely on their personal experiences.

11. How do I help students handle frustration before and after a forum discussion?

11. For a more personal touch, e-mail students who seem to be having major angst about diverse cultural content and inclusive instruction; encourage them to take a week and simply read other students' comments. Consider making this same exception for students who are dominating the discussion. Also, you can ask the entire class to refrain from writing for a week and just re-read the comments.

12. How do I recognize a "teachable moment" for assisting learners in respecting diversity?

12. A "teachable moment" is any moment where students are discussing, debating or even arguing about why diversity is so important. Other critical moments include students discussing their perception of clients' needs or even when they are grasping medical terminology and procedures. It is important for students to understand

and reflect upon those linguistic, social, intrapersonal, and even ethnic factors that influence their own learning. According to the Arizona State University Intergroup Relations Center (2001), one strong teachable moment is when students are allowed to talk openly about an instructor's statement that was misunderstood or perceived as inappropriate.

13. *How do I decide what culturally relevant skills and dispositions to assess?*

13. First, review where the course fits into the students' overall requirements for a degree and/or a license. On a piece of paper, jot down clinical skills and attitudes in one column and culturally relevant skills and attitudes in the other. Try to find similarities between the two lists. The similarities may serve as the criteria for assessing future culturally aware and culturally sensitive professionals. Don't forget to use certification and accreditation manuals and articles describing the nursing profession's multicultural goals.

14. *How can I assess diversity in learners?*

14. Require reflective writing assignments that ask students to explore a critical incident in their clinical experiences or in the classroom. Ask them to present what happened, how it worked, what research speaks to the facts and the results of the incident, and what social and cultural implications exist in the experience (Zeichner & Liston, 1987). Allow students to take on expert "diversity" roles. Ask half of the class to assume the role of expert (researching answers and disseminating information) and assign the role of inquirer (researching questions and presenting field-based incidents) to the other half.

15. *How can I assist learners to assess their own interaction with diversity?*

15. Ask students to evaluate assignments on the basis of new knowledge discovered, affirmation of ideas, and conflicts with various perspectives. Peer teaching is still one of the best ways to encourage and assess student knowledge. Pair students and require them to present their experiences as a teacher and a learner. Also, allow students to present together on different perspectives of the same issue. After the projects are completed, ask students to individually report on lessons learned about peer dynamics.

16. *What Web sites can provide culturally relevant information for students and for me as an instructor?*

16. Browse sites such as the Multicultural Pavilion for broad and specific information for self-scoring and classroom discussion. Another activity is Diversophy Online which may provoke inquiries into stereotyping and generalizations. If you want to learn more about the scholarship centered on diversity in higher education, check out

Diversity Web. There are plenty of general and discipline-specific online conversations about diversity that exist. Don't be afraid to be a diversity Web crawler!

17. Overall, what are the basic principles for assisting learners in a Web course to become culturally aware and culturally competent?

17. As you grapple with and succeed at online teaching and learning, be aware of the messages that you are sending. Consistently ask for students' feedback. Find a balance between interactivity and self-reflection. Also, keep a log of your goals, lessons learned, and your accomplishments as you integrate cultural awareness and culturally sensitive competency. View your course transformation as a process and not a product with a deadline. Above all, make your course a journey where in it lies reflection and effort from individuals and from the whole class.

RESOURCES

Arizona State University Intergroup Relations Center. (2001, August 2). *Classroom resources: Conflict de-escalation.* Retrieved September 18, 2002, from **http://www.asu.edu/provost/intergroup/resources/classconflict.html**

Association of American Colleges and Universities & University of Maryland, College Park. *Diversity Web: An interactive resource hub for higher education.* **http://www.diversityweb.org**

Gorski, P. *Multicultural Pavilion.* **http://curry.edschool.virginia.edu/go/multicultural**

Moore, G. S., Winograd, K., & Lange, D. (2001). *You can teach online: Building a creative environment.* Boston: McGraw-Hill.

Morey, A. I., & Kitano, M. K. (1996). *Multicultural course transformation in higher education: A broader truth.* New York: Allyn and Bacon.

Zeichner, K., & Liston, D. (1987). Teaching student teachers to reflect. *Harvard Educational Review, 57*(1), 23-48.

Section 9:
E-Quality: Evaluation, Accreditation, and Evidence for Best Practices

Educators, learners, administrators, accreditation agencies, parents, business partners, and nursing organizations are interested in knowing if e-learning "works." Will the quality be comparable to traditional learning? Who will assure the quality? Who will monitor the providers of online education? Who will accredit e-learning programs? What is the evidence for best practices in teaching and learning in online communities? In this unit you will learn about methods, strategies, and policies for assuring quality and continuous quality improvement in e-learning.

Chapter 29: *Strategies to Evaluate and Grade Learning*

1. What is involved in evaluating learning in e-learning courses?

1. As with traditional classroom-based courses, evaluation of learning in online courses is an important part of the teaching-learning process. And, as you do when evaluating learning outcomes in on-campus courses, you will

- design the course or module with clearly stated learning objectives outcomes/competencies;

- provide learning experiences and activities that give the learner an opportunity to activate the objectives/competencies;

- offer opportunities to practice and obtain feedback prior to evaluation;

- specify the behavior or product that the learner will produce to demonstrate that learning has occurred.

For the most part, evaluation strategies that work in the on-campus classroom (such as tests, portfolios, papers, concept maps, simulations) will also work in Web courses. In fact, the learning management system tools such as online testing, online gradebooks, and text editors make evaluation and grading much easier. The most important aspect of evaluation in online courses is to develop a course evaluation plan and share it with the learners at the beginning of the course.

2. What is a course evaluation plan?

2. A course evaluation plan is the overall guide to how you are going to evaluate learning, the strategies you are going to use, the work the learner must submit to indicate the learning outcomes are achieved, and the criteria for the "grades" or "pass-fail" indicators. For example, a plan might indicate the number of examinations for the course, the content to be mastered prior to taking the exam, the number of questions on the exam, the point value of the exam in relation to other evaluation strategies, and the date the exam will be administered. Once the course evaluation plan is established, it becomes the vehicle through which the educator communicates with learners how they will be evaluated and what weight and grade will be attributed to evaluation. A course evaluation plan is even more important in an online course; well developed and clearly stated evaluation plans minimize anxiety about what is expected in the course.

3. When should I evaluate and grade learners in online courses?

3. It is important to evaluate student learning on an ongoing basis. You may want to establish "check points" along the way.

Formative evaluation early in the course is important to e-learners, as they need information not only about how they are attaining learning outcomes, but also about how they are doing in the online learning community. Formative evaluation assists learners to chart their progress, and along with teaching feedback, assists them to attain outcomes. The testing and gradebook tools of the learning management system can assist you and the learners to keep track of milestones, such as completing a module, attaining mastery on an exam, or completing course activities.

Summative evaluation occurs at the end of the module or course. At this point the learner is ready to demonstrate attainment of course objectives.

Grading, unlike formative and summative feedback, is the value judgment about the learner's attainment of learning outcomes. The grading requirements should be clearly stated at the outset and activities for which "grades" (as opposed to formative or summative evaluation) will be assigned should be made clear to the learners.

4. What evaluation strategies work best in online courses?

4. Most of your favorite evaluation strategies will work in an online course, although some may require some adaptation or "work arounds." Here are a few evaluation strategies that work well and take advantage of the tools within the learning management software:

- **Tests.** You can use all types of tests, including essay, matching, and multiple choice, in online courses. You can use these tests for practice, mastery, and final evaluation. Be sure to select a learning management system and course tools to include the test authoring features you most commonly use.

- **Written work.** Written work such as diaries, reflection papers, written project papers, and one-minute summaries work well as formative or summative evaluation in online courses. Students can submit individual or group papers and post them in a public discussion forum or submit them as private e-mail or in a private forum where only the course facilitator/faculty will see the work. Peer feedback is a useful way for students to improve their written work prior to submitting it for grading.

- **Games, simulations, debates.** These strategies also work and provide variety and diversity to the evaluation plan. When using these strategies for evaluation (as opposed to teaching), be sure learners practice and have opportunities for feedback before using these for final evaluation.

- **Case studies, problems, or critical thinking activities.** These can be easily used as an evaluation by posting in the course discussion forum, sending as private e-mail, or using as an essay test. Learners can complete these evaluations as individuals or in groups by taking them as an essay test, as an e-mail response, or as a posting on the discussion board.

- **Discussion, participation, completion of learning activities.** Attainment of learning outcomes is clearly evident as the learner produces observable comments and completes assignments. Be sure to identify the grading criteria for what constitutes "A," "B," or "pass/fail" level work.

- **Portfolios.** Portfolios or other cumulative records of a body of work in a course can also be used in online courses. Learners can submit the portfolio electronically or by mail.

- **Posters.** An electronic "poster" presented as a PowerPoint presentation is an effective strategy for assessing the learner's ability to synthesize key points. Posters give students an opportunity to exercise creativity and demonstrate originality. Simple posters can be as effective as those with complex graphics, audio, or video.

5. How can I use the tools in a learning management system (LMS) to facilitate evaluation and grading?

5. Now you are thinking like an e-educator! Use those tools to your advantage. Here is a starter list of ideas:

- Simple test development, administration, grading, and record keeping using the testing and gradebook tools of a LMS (see Chapter 30 for more information).

- Use course e-mail when you want private responses, but keep submissions short, or you will have a lot of e-mail to grade!

- For group projects have students submit one paper or summary in the discussion forum. Use the discussion forum for one-minute summaries or reflection papers that summarize succinctly learning outcomes from complex assignments.

- Use rubrics and Classroom Assessment Techniques (CATs) to make evaluation simpler.

- Learn to use the word editing tools for giving feedback and grading papers. The learning curve is high, but worth it if you are going to be commenting on several drafts of a paper. Because this tool facilitates document sharing, learners can obtain feedback from classmates and colleagues as well as from the educator.

6. How do I evaluate and grade course participation?

6. A large portion of learning time in teacher-facilitated online courses is spent in course participation and discussion. Discussion is a way for both formative and summative evaluation and monitoring the development and use of critical thinking skills.

Evaluation standards or rubrics should be identified prior to the start of the course. Since so much time is spent in discussion (and as a way to encourage and reward high quality discussion), it is advisable to allocate sufficient amount of the grade to discussion. Some educators suggest awarding as much as 20 percent of the course grade for discussion and online learning activities.

Grading course participation is more accurate in online courses, as the discussion is visible and on record throughout the course. Thus, grading can be less subjective than in classroom courses where faculty give grades for classroom participation. It is important to keep the grading of course participation simplified in a course in which there is a lot of discussion. Using grading rubrics and Classroom Assessment Techniques are several ways to keep formative and summative evaluation and grading manageable.

7. What are grading rubrics?

7. A rubric is a scoring guide that establishes the criteria for grading. Rubrics specify gradations for quality, and, therefore, are differentiators that can be used to determine grades. Rubrics are useful because they clarify learning outcomes, establish expectations, communicate what is to be learned, and specify how grades will be assigned. Rubrics are authentic, real world and performance-based values that are compatible with the values of many health professions educators. Rubrics arc helpful in e-learning because they serve as guides for learners to monitor their work and that of their classmates. Rubrics can reduce the amount of time spent in evaluating student work because the student in the course and his/her classmates can improve the quality of the work to be evaluated prior to submitting the work for evaluation. E-learning courses lend themselves to using rubrics because of the public and collaborative nature of learning in the online community. Rubrics are useful in evaluating and grading discussion and course participation.

8. What are classroom assessment techniques?

8. Classroom Assessment Techniques (CATs) are short, easy to use strategies to assess learning as well as teaching and course effectiveness. CATs are learner-centered, teacher-directed, and context-specific techniques that can be used to gather information that can then be used to make modifications in teaching and learning. You may be familiar with popular CATs such as a "one-minute summary," "muddiest point," or "application cards." CATs work well in Web courses:

1. To assess prior knowledge (background probes)

2. As formative assessment

3. To determine how the course is going

4. As quick ways to assess learning for a lesson/module

5. To help students identify their own values, self awareness—CATs work well for "affective domain" types of learning—particularly since you lack the face-to-face sense of this

6. To determine learners' reactions to Web teaching/learning and learning activities

7. To manage time—yours and the students

When you use CATs in Web courses, follow the same principles for using CATs on the Web as you do in the classroom: plan carefully, test them before using them, give the learners feedback about the results, and use the findings to improve teaching, learning, or the course.

9. How do I evaluate and grade "attitudes" and other affective domain attributes?

9. Learning in nursing involves a significant component of affective domain learning such as recognizing the values and beliefs of self and others, acquiring values of the profession, socialization, professionalization, or acquiring cultural competence. Strategies that work well for evaluating affective domain attributes in e-learning

courses include values clarification exercises (pre/post check lists), portfolios, pre/post reflection statements, discussion boards, and case study discussions.

10. Can students evaluate each other?

10. Yes, students are a great source of feedback and evaluation for their classmates. Having students evaluate each other accomplishes several instructional goals. First, because students can read each others' comments on the discussion board, they can offer peer critique and provide suggestions to demonstrate their own critical thinking about each others' posting. Student evaluation of each other's work is also a way to develop professional values and responsibilities for peer review. Finally, the tools of e-learning facilitate collaborative group work, and educators can design collaborative work group experiences that provide opportunities for students to give feedback and evaluate each others' work in the context of the collaborative work group.

11. How do you inform students about their progress?

11. There are several ways of informing students about course progress. Progress reports can be public, in which case all course members can see the responses, and, thereby, learn from the comments, or private. *Public feedback* occurs as a response from the course facilitator or another classmate to student's comments in a discussion board or chat room. *Private evaluation* can occur in e-mail or gradebook comments accessible only to the student. As the person responsible for the evaluation plan within the course, be cautious about what information about course progress is public vs. private.

Most testing tools and e-course gradebooks have functions that can be set so the student can see instructor's comments or the grade on a test or assignment. Be sure to check for these functions and make decisions about how to set them so learners can follow their progress. Most students want to be able to keep track of their own progress, and the electronic gradebook makes this possible.

12. How will I know that it is really the learner who is doing the work?

12. How much security you impose when evaluating learning outcomes will depend on your own philosophy, the requirements of your institution, and the nature of the learning to be evaluated. There is a wide range of security options you can use. If you want to be absolutely certain the student is the one doing the work, you will need to have tightly controlled circumstances such as a heavily proctored testing center or classroom. Here students bring identification, leave all materials outside of the room, and take alternative forms of the exam. A less restrictive approach is to minimize the opportunity for students to misrepresent themselves and their work. Here are some suggestions (Other suggestions specific to online exams are discussed in Chapter 30):

- Establish expectations for academic honesty in the course. If the school or university or healthcare agency has academic honesty policies, be sure the learner is aware of them, and link to them or post them in the course.

- Learn about the students and their work and look for inconsistent patterns. Collaborate and communicate with colleagues, clinical faculty, and preceptors who know the students in a direct and personal way.

- Have proctors at locations convenient for the students.

- Set the Internet protocol (IP) address and check that the student is accessing the course from a consistent address.

- Spot check exam answers and compare them with other students and times at which they completed an online test.

- Use a variety of evaluation methods. Do not rely totally on tests or only written work as evaluation strategies.

- Use online services that scan students' written work for plagiarism.

Resources

Angelo, T., & Cross, K. P. (1993). *Classroom assessment techniques*. San Francisco: Jossey-Bass.

http://www.hcc.hawaii.edu/intranet/committees/FacDevCom/guidebk/teachtip/assess-1.htm

http://www.www.ntlf.com/htm/lib/bib/assess.htm

http://www.siue.edu/~deder/assess/catmain.html

http://edWeb.sdsu.edu/Webquest/rubrics/Weblessons.html

Chapter 30: *Online Testing*

1. *What is online testing? What can be tested online?*

1. Online testing is the administration of tests to learners using computer technology. This type of testing is typically accomplished by using server-based or Web-based programs. Depending on the program, there is a wide range of applicability for online testing including use of testing in formal classroom settings instead of paper-and-pencil testing, the demonstration of competency in knowledge-based content, and documentation of "mandatory" inservice program completion in institutions. Many programs also have test-bank capabilities.

2. *What is the difference between server-based and Web-based online testing?*

2. Server-based applications are typically reserved for a set number of computer workstations where the institution has disk space to run and house the testing program. A local area network (LAN) is used to provide a distribution network to the computers that it serves. Web-based testing uses the World Wide Web, through use of a Web browser, to deliver the test. Either type of testing may be desirable depending on the resources available to the institution.

3. *Why is there a "push" for online testing?*

3. There are several reasons why online testing has increased in popularity. One is that the national licensure exam (NCLEX-RN) for nurses has become computerized and certification exams in nursing specialties are moving in this direction. Nursing education programs want students to become comfortable with technology prior to taking the national exam, and online testing is one means to achieve that goal. Another reason for the increase in online testing is to deliver a cost-effective means for showing competency in an individual. A number of programs are available to institutions, or are being developed in-house, that test employees' competencies without requiring another employee to hand grade each test. Typically online testing programs come with some sort of reporting mechanism to assist in the record-keeping process. Finally, many nursing programs have set information technology competencies for their graduates. Online testing is one means to show competency in that area.

4. *What types of questions may be used in online testing?*

4. The types of questions available may vary among programs, but a robust learning management system will offer a full range of question options including true-false, multiple choice, matching, multiple multiples (more than one correct answer), short answer, and essay.

5. Is there any evidence in support of online testing?

5. One study demonstrated a significant difference in practice test scores in a convenience sample of 42 students in an undergraduate pharmacology course (Rossignol & Scollin, 2001). The group of students who took the practice tests by computer demonstrated higher test scores. Students in this study reported they would feel more comfortable taking the licensure (NCLEX-RN) examination. In another study computerized testing in a convenience sample of 127 undergraduate nursing students was assessed (Bloom & Trice, 1997). Computerized testing groups performed the same or better on tests when compared to groups taking paper-and-pencil tests. In the long run, learners taking computer-based tests have similar scores to those taking conventional tests (Wise & Plake, 1990).

6. What are the major advantages of online testing?

6. One of the major advantages is that online testing, especially in a Web-based environment, is accessible to many different audiences in different locations. Another advantage, as described above, is that online testing may be beneficial to institutions that require competency testing and that currently use employees to hand grade tests. Some online testing programs allow for immediate feedback to be given to the examinee, and allow examinees to take the test until they achieve competency without multiple paper copies of the test. In some cases, online testing allows for convenient retrieval of results without taking the test or answer sheets to a different location for analysis. Often, online testing programs provide immediate reports for analysis of results, and some programs will automatically calculate the exam statistics right after the test.

7. What are the major barriers to online testing?

7. The most significant barrier to online testing is the cost of human and technical resources. Although online testing may lower human resource costs by reducing hand grading, support is needed throughout the online testing process. In addition, computer workstations must be adequate in number and computing capability to support online testing. The examinee must have the necessary computer skills to navigate through the program. Finally, test security is an issue for some online testing programs.

8. When is online testing appropriate and when is it not appropriate?

8. Online testing is appropriate when learners desire immediate feedback and the instructors wish to decrease the resources associated with grading and record keeping. Online testing is not appropriate for a secure

test when adequate instructor supervision is not available. Online testing can also be counter productive in largely essay tests where individuals may not have adequate keyboarding skills.

9. What are the aspects of online testing that learners enjoy the most?

9. This depends on the focus of the online test, but learners seem to value the immediate feedback on their performance. In addition, for some online testing programs, the rationale for answers can be provided at the end of the test. Students who take online tests during their educational programs also appreciate becoming comfortable with computer testing before they take a licensure or certification examination.

10. What are the aspects of online testing that learners find difficult?

10. Clearly the online format, specifically computer screens, is a different context for test taking. Most learners have tested through traditional paper-and-pencil examinations, and a change to online testing initially causes some discomfort. One of the most common complaints from learners is that they cannot write on the tests, a strategy often used to help learners think through a question and possible answers. To combat that issue, some instructors allow the students to use a piece of paper. Finally, learners may find use of computers for testing to be an uncomfortable experience because it is unfamiliar. Learners are already stressed by the fact they are being evaluated, and the change in the delivery of the evaluation tool is sometimes an issue.

11. What resources are needed to do online testing?

11. Unless the institution has the capability of developing an online testing program, it will have to be purchased from a vendor. The costs vary depending upon the level of complexity, capabilities, and format of the program. In addition, as newer versions of the program are released, there may be a need to upgrade the program. The human resources required for online testing may be extensive. Someone who is familiar with online products will need to make the decision on which program to purchase. If that person does not exist within the institution, paid consultants may be needed to facilitate the process. Significant human resources will be needed to install, implement, and train individuals for the use of the program. Training includes appropriate education for those facilitating online testing as well as training for the examinees. There must also be adequate human support for trouble-shooting throughout program usage. Investment in computer workstations may also be necessary, especially if the testing is to be done onsite. Workstations must be able to minimally meet the program specifications for operation.

12. What types of products are available to assist with online testing?

12. An excellent comparative review of computerized test development software was published in *Computers in Nursing* (Kirkpatrick et al., 2000). Nine programs were reviewed on the following traits: security, pedagogical capabilities, test design, and administration procedures. Not only does the review provide detailed descriptions of the program, but it also provides criteria used to evaluate the program that others may use as well.

13. What are the major pitfalls that can happen during online testing and how can I avoid them?

13. The nightmare of any instructor is that a test is scheduled for a specific time period in a specific location, and the test does not come up for the learner, or it disappears while the learner is taking the test. Testing failures may occur for the following reasons: 1) there is a server problem on which the program is housed; 2) there is a computer workstation problem; and/or 3) the program was not set up by the instructor properly. For example, the date or time for release to the user was not set properly. It is important to know the capability and stability of the server before the initiation of online testing.

While in the process of purchasing a program, ask the vendor for a test run using the server and computer workstations. Some programs allow you to set up a "dry run" of the test before it is made available to learners. Adequate computer support is necessary to ensure the proper functioning of computer workstations. Quality workstations are a critical investment if the implementation of online testing is desired. Instituting online testing is a learning adventure for the instructor as well. Most instructors who do online testing have learned the intricacies of the programs by making mistakes in setting up the test. To avoid problems during the actual test, it is strongly advised to run a simulated test before implementation. In summary, planning and implementing a simulated test before the actual testing can avoid most of the pitfalls.

14. What are the security issues with online testing? How do they compare with paper-and-pencil testing?

14. The three largest threats to online testing are 1) hacking into a test, 2) downloading and sharing the test, and 3) printing of a test. Unfortunately, there may be very little control over these activities. If test security is a major issue for the testing situation, special attention should be paid to those features when selecting a program.

Online tests delivered through a specific server and that are not Web-based may provide for the best security. The drawback is limited access to computers because of the reach of the server. If the testing to be implemented will only be given onsite, this may be the best option. Web-based testing provides for the greatest access—learners may access a Web-based program through any computer that has Internet access. The most significant security threats are through this means. While many people will not attempt to break security through "hacking" into a test that is institution specific, there is always that possibility. Web browsers such as Netscape® and Microsoft Explorer®, have a menu bar that allows the program, in this case, the test, to be downloaded and/or printed. Further, controlling the printing in a specific cluster of computers may be possible, but if the computers are networked to printers outside of the cluster, the learner may be able to print to another computer without the instructor's knowledge.

15. How can I maintain test security?

15. The best ways to maintain test security are to: 1) select an online testing program that allows the type of security desired; 2) use all of the security features available in the program; and 3) provide proctoring during testing. If a high-level security system were desired, the following features would be beneficial:

- Login with username and password for each learner

- High security feature (lock and key) with Web-based programs

- Scrambling ability for test questions and test answers, so each user has a unique test

- Accessibility features allowing the instructor to turn off and turn on the test at certain dates and times, and controlling testing time

- Feedback features allowing a variety of feedback from full question text and correct answer, to just the correct number of items, to no feedback at all.

In some instances when the test is being administered at different times to different groups, high-level security is not always possible for the same reasons it would not be possible in a traditional paper-and-pencil exam. To further enhance security, the test should be given at the same time to all learners and the test should be proctored.

16. How will I know the appropriate learners are taking the test?

16. There are two main ways to ensure that the learners who should take the test are the learners who are actually taking the test: 1) require a login with a username and password; and 2) proctor the exam requiring all learners to be in attendance in the same computer cluster. If it is a large group where the instructor does not know the learners, similar techniques to those used in paper-and-pencil exams should be added. The most common technique is checking learner identification prior to the start of the test.

If the test is being given at different times and may be taken on the learner's own computer, assurance of appropriate ethical behavior is much harder to monitor. A username and password are still the best means, but the instructor might also consider using a statement at the beginning of the exam where test-takers attest that they are, indeed, the right test-taker. Learners can also be required to go to testing centers in their community where proctors can verify student identity and monitor the test taking.

17. How can I use online tests and surveys for formative evaluation?

17. Formative evaluation occurs during the course of a learning event or program. Online tests for the purposes of formative evaluation can be used to help prepare the learner for a particular module, class session, and pre-testing. Quizzes may be used as a means to prepare learners prior to a class and may be either graded or ungraded. In some instances, the instructor may wish the learner to achieve a certain grade level before class, even if it means multiple attempts at the quiz. Instructors may also wish to pose questions to students as a means for reflection prior to class to facilitate a class session. Tests may also be given prior to and after covered content to measure what learners have gained as a result of classroom intervention.

18. How can I use online tests and surveys to obtain feedback from students to improve the course? Can I administer a test or survey and protect the learner's anonymity?

18. Online tests and surveys may be used to gain feedback from students about a variety of classroom strategies for the purposes of course improvement. The types of questions range from Likert-type questions to open-ended questions. The major issue with obtaining feedback about a course is protecting the learner's identity. While there are programs available allowing the instructor to ensure anonymity, there are also programs that do not. If you are using a program that requires a username and password to log into the test or survey, learner responses are traceable. Many programs will also record the IP address, or the specific computer from which the response was generated. However, the responses are often not listed with the IP address. If it is the case that users could be traced, there should be a data steward who is not the instructor. A data steward is an individual in charge of the program and its operations. Typically, learners who use programs that require logging in should be directed that the only situation where their responses will be traced is in the instance of a threatening response.

19. What type of grading/reporting features should I look for in an online testing program?

19. In general, the most sophisticated grading/reporting features reasonably needed should be selected. Many programs allow the instructor to determine the number of points each question will be worth and will calculate the learner's grade accordingly. Some programs will grade short answer questions by looking for key words or performing a word match. Grade reports should list the username, the grade (with the ability to review the responses of each learner's test), the time required, and the IP address. If a record-keeping system is desired, a program with an integrative gradebook allowing for the transfer of the testing grades is highly beneficial. Reports should also generate statistics about the test. There are a variety of statistics available:

- Percentage of learners selecting response per response

- Upper third versus lower third (shows how the upper third of the class, as determined by overall test score, performed on a particular question)

- Mean, median, mode, standard deviation

- Reliability measures

20. What are electronic gradebooks and how are they used?

20. Electronic gradebooks are a means for record keeping of tests, competencies, or the results of testing on the so called mandatory education programs used by most healthcare agencies. Online testing does not have to be done to use an electronic gradebook; however, many online testing programs also have the capability for electronic gradebooks. Electronic gradebooks typically allow learners to access their grades using their username and password.

RESOURCES

Bloom, K. C., & Trice, L. B. (1997). The efficacy of individualized computerized testing in nursing education. *Computers in Nursing, 15*(2), 82–88.

Kirkpatrick, J. M., Billings, D. M., Hodson Carlton, K., Cummings, R. B., Dorner, J., Jeffries, P. R., et al. (2000). Computerized test development software: A comparative review updated. *Computers in Nursing, 18*(2), 72–86.

Rossignol, M., & Scollin, P. (2001). Piloting use of computerized practice tests. *Computers in Nursing, 19*(5), 206–212.

Wise, S. L., & Plake, B. B. (1990). Computer-based testing system. *Measurement and Evaluation in Counseling and Development, 23*(4), 3–10.

Chapter 31: Evaluation of Online Courses

1. What is involved in evaluating online courses?

1. As with the development of any course, it is important to evaluate the course design, structure, teaching and learning activities, and the evaluation plan. When evaluating online courses, however, it is also necessary to evaluate the graphic design, the user interfaces, learners' use and appropriateness of the collaborative work tools, design of learning activities, consideration for varying learning styles as well as the ease with which the learner can navigate within the course.

2. When should I evaluate the course?

2. Because developing and teaching in online courses are new for most educators and learners, it is important to evaluate the course frequently. Ideally, the course should be fully evaluated during the design process with a few learners (pilot testing), and while the course is offered the first time (field/usability testing). Data from pilot testing and field testing will inform decisions for awarding contact hours, estimating the time it is taking the learners to complete the course, and to guide course revision. When the course is offered on a regular basis, course evaluation procedures can be simplified.

3. What is a pilot test?

3. A pilot test is a test of how well the course works during its development. Pilot testing is a formal instructional design procedure and involves obtaining peer review of the course content and teaching and evaluation strategies as well as determining how well the course works for the learners. Pilot testing uses a small (3 to 5) group of a range of the members of the "target audience," thus large groups of learners are not at risk for enrolling in an ineffective course. While conducting a pilot test for an academic course is ideal, pilot tests are essential for continuing education modules/courses in order to determine the number of contact hours to award. Pilot tests provide immediate data for course revision and save time and effort in course redesign.

4. How do I conduct a pilot test?

4. Pilot tests are conducted by members of the user audience such as students, registered nurses, or nurses in a specialty practice. You should identify three to five learners who will be similar to those who will be taking the course. Seek diversity in this group; for example, learners from a variety of geographic areas, varying experience with using computers, or from different educational settings. If possible, provide a modest

honorarium or a complimentary registration at a continuing education offering to reward the participants for their time. Ask the learners to complete the course and provide feedback about what is going well and where the "rough spots" are. Provide a checklist for ease of course review.

The pilot test also includes peer review of the course content and learning activities. Here you will ask a colleague or two to review the course for content accuracy, appropriateness of the level of the content for the learner, the suitability of the learning activities, and the time expectations for the learner based on the course structure (credit hours or estimated contact hours). Again, a checklist can guide the reviewer and simplify data analysis.

5. What is a field test?

5. A field test, or usability test, involves a larger number of participants, and in practicality, is usually the first offering of a course. For the field test you will gather detailed information about how the course works for both you and the learners.

6. How do I conduct a field test?

6. To conduct a field test, you will use the course under the conditions in which the learners for which it is intended will normally use it. You will follow the learners from registration through course completion. Solicit feedback often; use course tools to gather data anonymously; ask learners what is working and what is not. Be open to changing the course mid-stream if something is not going well. The end-of-course evaluation instruments should have sufficient detail so you are collecting significant information from the learners. It may also be helpful to keep a journal of your impressions of what is working and what needs to be changed. If practical and useful, make the changes immediately so you do not forget them for the next course offering.

7. From whom shall I gather information about a course?

7. It is helpful to obtain feedback about the course design and usability from as many sources as are practical. *You* will be a significant source of data—keep a diary, log, notes or a reflection paper about how the course is going and what revisions should be included the next time the course is offered.

Learners will also provide helpful feedback. As you teach the course, observe how students react, what presents them with difficulty, and where they are confused. At the end of the course, ask them to be candid with their comments and assure them their suggestions are anonymous (and be sure they are!) and will be used to improve the course design and structure.

Feedback from an *instructional designer or graphic artist* also can be helpful. If you have access to a Web course design team or an office of instructional support, contact them and ask them to review the course. The design team may also have a course evaluation instrument that could be used to guide review of the course.

8. What about peer review of Web courses?

8. Peer review is a process by which a colleague with similar background and experience (in other words, a peer!) reviews a course. The peer should be someone who has developed and taught in a Web course and has sufficient expertise to provide a helpful review. Peer review is a common activity in colleges and universities with tenure and promotion procedures, as peer review is one way of gathering information to support promotion and tenure in the area of teaching. Peer review is best conducted after field testing and teaching the course once or twice. It usually works well to invite the peer reviewer into the course after the course is well underway so the peer reviewer can see what is going on with the teaching and learning activities. Be sure to request permission from the course participants to have a guest peer reviewer in the course.

9. Where can I find a peer reviewer for a course?

9. Colleagues who are teaching Web courses similar to yours are ideal peer reviewers. Colleagues from other disciplines who have experience with developing and teaching in Web courses (technically this is a "colleague" as opposed to a true "peer") can provide similar and equally helpful information about the course design and the teaching and learning activities, if not about the content. Instructional support offices that are supporting Web courses at healthcare agencies or colleges and universities are other potential sources for course review.

10. Who will be interested in the results of the course evaluation?

10. Internal and external audiences are interested in the results of evaluations of Web courses. You, as course faculty, are the most important recipient of the course evaluation findings, as you are the one who will be making changes, and submitting the results for merit review or promotion or tenure review. Keep a "teaching portfolio" of your course development work.

Your supervisor or department chair will be interested in knowing about the course and its success. Be sure to alert him/her to the fact that you are teaching a Web course for the first time and are testing new ways of teaching. Provide a context for interpreting the findings. Combine your reflections with those of the learners and peers to give a 360° picture of course development.

Findings from Web course evaluations will also be useful to administrators who are monitoring the success of online courses and programs. External audiences such as accrediting agencies, parents of students, or professional nursing organizations are carefully following the success of online courses, and your results will assist in informing their perceptions and subsequent decisions. Finally, do not forget about your colleagues who are also developing Web courses and may benefit from an article in the nursing literature about your experiences and findings!

RESOURCES

Cobb, K., Billings, D., Mays, R., & Canty-Mitchell, J. (2001). Peer review of Web based courses in nursing. *Nurse Educator*, 26(6), 274–279.

Institute for Higher Education Policy. (2000). Quality on the line: Benchmarks for success in Internet-based distance education. Washington, DC: Author.

Chapter 32: Benchmarking Best Practices E-Learning

1. What is benchmarking?

1. In its earliest form, benchmarking was developed by primitive craftsmen who marked their workbenches to ensure an easy, repeatable way of measuring materials for cutting to a given length. Since the early 1980s, benchmarking has been used extensively by the business sector as a quality improvement tool for allowing organizations to compare themselves with the best. It is a technique used to help organizations to become as good as or better than the best in their class. Camp (1995) defined benchmarking as a search for implementation of best practices. Benchmarking is more than just gathering data. It involves adapting a new approach of continually questioning how processes are performed, seeking out best practices, and implementing new models of operation. Although benchmarking has received much attention in the business world for the last two decades, only recently is it advancing in the education arena.

2. What are "Best Practices"?

2. Best practices are documented strategies or tactics employed by highly successful organizations. Because of the organization's drive for excellence, these practices have been implemented and perfected to make them most admired by others. These strategies or tactics are supported by research or evidence to illustrate their achievement. Best practices in education are strategies used to produce good teaching and learning outcomes including customer satisfaction. The most widely used good practices in post-secondary education are those defined by Chickering and Gamson (1987) and later by Chickering and Ehrmann (1996).

3. Are there different types of benchmarking?

3. There are several different types of benchmarking, and this often adds to the confusion about the process. Camp (1989) proposed the first basic taxonomy of best practice benchmarking types, and these have been adopted and adapted by many authors following him; however, most agree that these unique types actually do fit the basic four as projected by Camp: internal, competitive, functional, and generic. Each of the types focuses on identifying, observing, measuring, and learning from best practices.

Internal benchmarking focuses primarily on in-house practices or processes across different departments or functions.

Competitive benchmarking seeks to identify comparable measures with others considered to be direct competitors. It looks to identify practice performance gaps with competitors. Competitive benchmarking can be internal or external.

Functional benchmarking makes comparisons with organizations from the same sector, using similar processes.

Generic benchmarking looks to identify and transfer innovative best practices from one industry to another. This type of benchmarking entices organizations to widen their benchmarking activities to include partners from different sectors.

4. Is benchmarking applicable to higher education?

4. Because of its reliance on hard data and research methodology, benchmarking is especially suited for institutions of higher education. Benchmarking can significantly affect the effectiveness of higher education by providing assistance in reaching strategic goals. The process of benchmarking helps overcome resistance to change, provides structure for external evaluation, and creates new networks of communication among schools where valuable information and experiences can be shared. It is viewed by most as a positive process that provides objective measurements for baselining, goal setting, and improvement tracking, which can lead to innovations, improved operations, and customer satisfaction. Despite the majority of positive recommendations for using benchmarking and successful examples of its current use, benchmarking processes in higher education have been slow to spread. Demands for accountability along with new tools and new strategies are swiftly changing that market sector.

5. Who should benchmark?

5. Anyone interested in an objective basis for improving operational performance by exploring best practices in other organizations should consider benchmarking. A review of the literature finds independent and group benchmarking studies being conducted at a variety of higher education institutions. Benchmarking is applicable for both administrators and faculty to improve organizational or teaching practices. Since online courses/programs are relatively new to higher education, any institution teaching such courses should consider benchmarking in order to establish and promote best practices in online learning communities.

6. When should you benchmark?

6. Before beginning a benchmarking study, an institution should decide if benchmarking is the correct quality improvement tool for the situation. Benchmarking should be used as a quality improvement tool any time an institution is interested in improving processes or staying competitive. As with other quality concepts, benchmarking should be integrated into the fundamental operations of the organization. It should be an ongoing process that establishes baseline information and collects data longitudinally and systematically. Then, the data should be used for monitoring, tracking, and making quality improvements.

7. How do I benchmark?

7. After you determine the processes or activities selected for analysis, the appropriate personnel to conduct the study should be chosen. These individuals should have a working knowledge of the area undergoing the benchmarking analysis. An institution can take part in an externally sponsored benchmarking project with predefined objectives, such as the Evaluating Educational Uses of the Web in Nursing (EEUWIN), or it can conduct a project on its own or with the assistance of a consultant. Information on potential benchmarking studies and partners is available through **http://www.tltgroup.org/programs/ftools.html**. Once the benchmarking data are collected and analyzed, they can be distributed in a benchmarking report internally within the institution and externally to the benchmarking partners for implementation of improved processes.

8. Why should I benchmark?

8. Benchmarking provides a powerful approach for institutions to spot strengths and gaps in their organizational practices and to identify proven practices for enhanced performance. Benchmarking data and real world experiences help guide institutions in making decisions about new or revised initiatives. It provides a focal point for sharing and discussing central issues and exploring practices that work. Benchmarking is catching on in higher education and is being supported by national accrediting agencies. New tools and new strategies including new technologies are making this process easier to incorporate into everyday business practices.

9. What are the steps in benchmarking?

9. The first step in the benchmarking process is to determine what to benchmark. Think about the stakeholders and what they may want to learn or need to learn about e-learning. It is at this stage that evaluation models, such

as the one proposed by the Flashlight Program, should be used to provide a framework for the study (Ehrmann & Zuniga, 1997). The variables in the Flashlight triad model include Outcomes, Educational Best Practices, and Use of Technology.

The second step is to enlist benchmarking partners and refine the mapping process. Determining the questions to be addressed and narrowing the focus of the study are the most important and time-consuming aspects of the process. The framework selected above assists with this process.

The third step is to develop a survey instrument. The Flashlight Current Student Inventory (CSI) provides a starting point in the design of the instrument. The CSI consists of over 500 survey items and interview questions indexed by technology and by educational issues, from which evaluators can choose to create their own study. Billings, Connors, and Skiba (2001) collaborated with the Flashlight Program team to develop and test the EEUWIN instrument specifically designed to benchmark best practices in online nursing courses.

The fourth step is to gather the performance data. Before doing this, remember to check to see what the institution's policies are in relation to use of human subjects. The EEUWIN instrument is available for benchmarking purposes on the Web through the Flashlight Program. For more information, contact **Flashlight@tltgroup.org** or visit **http://www.tltgroup.org/programs/ftools.html**.

The fifth step is analyzing performance by comparing practices and outcomes from different organizations against your own.

The final step is dissemination of the information to stakeholders for quality improvement.

10. How do I choose a framework or model for benchmarking?

10. The best way to choose a model or framework for your study is to first determine what it is that you want to know about e-learning. Then, review the literature to search for models or frameworks that support your thinking. You might want to expand these models or blend several models, perhaps from different disciplines, to develop and evaluate your own framework. For the purpose of benchmarking, you will want to keep the model simple so that you can demonstrate evidence to support the model and have consensus across institutions as to what is important in the model. You will find that different educational institutions will want to know similar things about the uses of technology in teaching and learning.

11. Where can I find benchmarking instruments?

11. Several national groups are leading efforts to develop and implement common frameworks that guide assessment of quality, cost, and outcomes of technology enabled courses and programs. The EEUWIN instrument mentioned above is one example. Another is the National Study of Student Engagement (NSSE) (**http://www.tltgroup.org/programs/ftools.html**). A literature search as well as a Web search can lead you to other benchmarking instruments.

12. Can I develop my own benchmarking instrument?

12. Yes, you can develop your own benchmarking instrument; however, if you are starting from scratch you will need to be sure that the instrument is psychometrically sound. Designing the measurement tool using the psychometric theory of instrumentation may take some valuable time. Remember, you don't want to reinvent the wheel. Starting with an instrument such as the Current Student Inventory (CSI) or using a standardized instrument may be a more efficient and effective way to proceed. You will still want to do some validity and reliability testing with your sample; however, validity and reliability have been previously established for these instruments and that should make your job easier.

13. How do I choose benchmarks?

13. Benchmarks are selected according to the strengths and weaknesses of the organization. Pinpoint strategic performance targets that are not being achieved and processes that appear to have improvement potential. Select the processes that are perceived as most in need of improvement. Care must be taken to ensure that the processes selected for improvement will actually yield the greatest benefits in terms of costs and implementation of strategies for change. Once you have identified processes in need of change, start looking for suitable benchmarking partners willing to share their experiences in relation to best practices in these processes. Benchmarking partners should include institutions similar to your own as well as institutions you consider to be your greatest competitors.

14. How can benchmarking ensure and enhance quality?

14. Benchmarking is a quality improvement technique that begins by recognizing best practices in other organizations and ends by learning how to match or surpass

229

those best practices. The benchmarking results are used to identify, understand, and adapt outstanding practices from other organizations to help the study sponsors improve their own organizations. The benefits are realized when organizations employ the benchmarking recommendations to analyze performance measures and make changes in the processes under study. Best practice benchmarks give the organization a goal or target to work toward. The charts and graphs allow you to readily spot strengths and gaps in performance and to track performance over time.

15. What does it cost to benchmark?

15. Benchmarking costs vary according to the different packages that are available through the Flashlight Program or other benchmarking services, the size of the institution, and the extensiveness of the study. Generally, the prices are cheaper if you are a member of the organization or network sponsoring the benchmarking project. A conservative estimate for average bench-marking activities for any one institution is in the range of $8,000 to $12,000 per year. In addition to funds for membership and toolkits, benchmarking requires a commitment of resources in terms of time for developing, implementing, and maintaining the benchmarking program. However, if an institution is serious about best practice quality improvement efforts, this is time and money well spent.

16. How do I use benchmarking data?

16. Benchmarking provides useful and relevant data for quality improvement in e-learning. Results can be used by administrators, individual faculty, instructional designers, and support staff to enhance or improve processes. First and foremost, the results can be used by individual faculty and/or instructional designers to strengthen and improve the teaching and learning strategies to support best practices. The benchmarking results provide a wealth of information about students' perceptions of their Web-based courses. These benchmarks encourage faculty to design Web courses with the educational practices supported by evidence-based research. Benchmarking results also allow administrators to apply the data in terms of administrative processes and practices that support technology-based learning. Using these data, better decisions can be made about technology, support services, and overall program outcomes needed to provide quality e-learning and to stay competitive in the marketplace.

RESOURCES

Billings, D. M. (2000). Framework for assessing outcomes and practices in Web-based courses in nursing. *Journal of Nursing Education, 39*(2), 60–67.

Billings, D. M., Connors, H. R., & Skiba, D. J. (2001). Benchmarking best practices in nursing Web-based courses. *Advances in Nursing Science, 23*(3), 41–52.

Camp, R. C. (1995). *Benchmarking: Finding and implementing best practices.* Milwaukee, WI: ASQC Quality Press.

Camp, R. C. (1989). *Benchmarking: The search for industry best practices that lead to superior performance.* Milwaukee, WI: ASQC Quality Press.

Chickering, A. W., & Ehrmann, S. (1996). *Implementing the seven principles: Technology as lever.* Retrieved February 4, 2002, from **http://www.tltgroup.org/programs/seven.html**

Chickering, A. W., & Gamson, Z. F. (1987). Seven principles for good practices in undergraduate education. *AAHE Bulletin, 39*(7), 3–6.

Ehrmann, S. C., & Zuniga, R. E. (1997). *The flashlight evaluation handbook.* Washington, DC: Corporation for Public Broadcasting.

Chapter 33: *Developing Courses for CE: Accreditation Issues*

1. What is accreditation?

1. Accreditation is any form of independent review of educational programs for the purpose of helping to establish that the learning offered is of a uniform and sound quality.

2. Why is accreditation important?

2. Accreditation is important when a public record of learning that will be widely accepted by employers, professional associations, and other colleges and universities is required. Accreditation is particularly important for e-learning courses and programs to assure consumers of course credibility and quality.

3. What kind of accreditation should I look for?

3. In the United States the most widely recognized form of accreditation for degree-granting programs comes from the regional accreditation boards. When people ask if you have attended an "accredited university" in the United States, they usually mean a regionally accredited university.

4. What about accreditation for nursing schools?

4. Nursing schools may also be accredited by state accrediting agencies as well as professional nursing organizations such as the National League for Nursing Accreditation Commission (NLNAC) and the Commission on Collegiate Nursing Education (CCNE) of the American Association of Colleges of Nursing (AACN). These organizations, composed of peers, establish standards for review of educational programs. For example, curriculum, faculty, resources, evaluation plan, quality of students admitted, and graduation rates are used to assure the quality of on-campus as well as Web courses.

5. If a university is accredited through one of the regional accreditation boards, does that mean its online courses are automatically accredited?

5. It is likely that any online course offered by an accredited "brick and mortar" university will be accredited, but it is not certain. It is important to ask about accreditation before registering for any online course. If the university is a totally virtual one without a "brick and mortar" presence, it is crucial to check carefully into its accreditation. If the university is not accredited by one of the six regional accreditation boards, then other accredited universities do not recognize any accreditation it may claim. Four virtual universities that are currently accredited by one of the six regional accreditation boards are Capella University at **www.capellauniversity.edu**, Walden University at **www.waldenu.edu**, University of Phoenix at **www.phoenix.edu**, and Jones University at **www.jonesinternational.edu**.

6. Are other types of accreditation recognized in the United States?

6. The Distance Education and Training Council (DETC) is a nationally recognized accreditation agency for distance learning colleges. The DETC also accredits institutions that sponsor home study programs of all kinds. However, credits and degrees earned at DETC colleges are not yet widely accepted in transfer by regionally accredited colleges.

Sometimes academic departments within colleges and universities seek special accreditation for their programs. Careers regulated by state or national licensing boards may require students to attend college departments that hold special accreditation. Teachers may be required to earn their education degrees from colleges whose education departments are accredited by the National Council for Accreditation of Teacher Education. Lawyers may be required to hold degrees from law schools that are accredited by the American Bar Association.

7. What are the principles of good practice for electronically offered academic degree and certificate programs?

7.
- Each program of study results in learning outcomes appropriate to the rigor and breadth of the degree or certificate awarded.

- An electronically offered degree or certificate program is coherent and complete.

- The program provides for appropriate real-time or delayed interaction between faculty and students and among students.

- Qualified faculty provide appropriate oversight of the program offered electronically.

- The program is consistent with the institution's role and mission.

- Review and approval processes ensure the appropriateness of the technology being used to meet the program's objectives.

- The program provides faculty support services specifically related to teaching via an electronic system.

- The program provides training for faculty who teach via the use of technology.

- The program ensures that appropriate learning resources are available to students.

- The program provides students with clear, complete, and timely information on the curriculum, course and degree requirements, nature of faculty/student interaction, assumptions about technological competence and skills, technical equipment requirements, availability of academic support services and financial aid resources, and costs and payment policies.

- Enrolled students have reasonable and adequate access to the range of student services appropriate to support their learning.

- Accepted students have the background, knowledge, and technical skills needed to undertake the program.

- Advertising, recruiting, and admissions materials clearly and accurately represent the program and the services available.

- Policies for faculty evaluation include appropriate consideration of teaching and scholarly activities related to electronically offered programs.

- The institution demonstrates a commitment to ongoing support, both financial and technical, and to continuation of the program for a period sufficient to enable students to complete a degree/certificate.

- The institution evaluates the program's educational effectiveness, including assessments of student learning outcomes, student retention, and student and faculty satisfaction. Students have access to such program evaluation data.

- The institution provides for assessment and documentation of student achievement in each course and at completion of the program.

8. What issues should be addressed in an organization's distance education policy?

8. Issues to be addressed by the institution's intellectual property policies should include:

- ownership of distance education courses

- institutional and faculty rights and responsibilities after a course is created

- faculty compensation

- teaching load and faculty acceptance

- student access and privacy

- potential liabilities associated with distance education courses (including copyright infringement liability)

- accreditation and approvals beyond state and national borders

9. How is an online course approved for professional continuing education hours?

9. An online course must meet the same criteria required for traditional courses. Many professional organizations set their own required standards in order for an online course to qualify for their specific hours. For example, the American Nurses Credentialing Center (ANCC) sets all requirements for courses to be approved for nursing continuing education hours. Physicians, lawyers, social workers, respiratory therapists, and pharmacists each have set criteria to qualify for their specific professional hours.

10. What kinds of online courses can be approved for professional continuing education hours?

10. Any online course that meets ANCC and state criteria can be approved for nursing contact hours. For nurses, the contact hours must be provided by an ANCC-accredited provider, approved by an ANCC-accredited approver, or approved by a state board of nursing. Programs for physicians, lawyers, respiratory therapists, social workers, and pharmacists may also have professional continuing education hours approved if the program meets that profession's specific criteria.

11. What are the standards that must be met in order to qualify for professional continuing education hours?

11. Nursing continuing education is defined by the ANCC as "systematic professional learning experiences designed to augment the knowledge, skills, and attitudes of nurses and therefore enrich the nurses' contributions to quality health care and their pursuit of professional career goals." (ANCC, **http://www.nursingworld.org/ancc/accred/accrdorg/appd.htm** on 5/22/02)

ANCC has specific criteria that must be met before an educational activity can be awarded nursing contact hours:

- The educational activity needs to enrich the nurse's contribution to health care.

- At least one nurse must be involved in the planning and one must have at least a BSN.

- The activity meets demonstrated educational needs of the participants.

- The purpose/goal of the learning activity is supported by its educational design.

- Educational objectives measure the expected outcomes for the learner.

- Learning objectives match the content presented.

- The time frame must be appropriate for the objectives and content.

- Presenters have knowledge and expertise in the content area.

- Presenters take an active part in developing their presentation.

- A biographical data form or curriculum vitae is provided by each presenter and planner.

- Teaching strategies match the objectives and content to be presented.

- Each participant has an opportunity to complete an evaluation that measures how well the objectives were met and the presentation content and effectiveness of teaching strategies. Evaluation of online offerings should include usability, clarity, and effectiveness of Web page design and links, and clarity of directions.

The following content does NOT qualify for nursing continuing education in most states:

- Information intended for the general public (e.g., non healthcare professionals)

- Information taught in basic or generic nursing education programs

- Preparation for or teaching a class

- Orientation—content referencing agency-specific information; role expectations

- For a specific work setting

- Inservice content to increase competency in fulfilling assigned responsibilities, such as single purpose equipment oriented briefings

- Activities that promote a product

To determine if other professions can be approved to receive their profession's approved continuing education hours, contact the following organizations for specific approval criteria:

- Physicians: ACCME (Accreditation Council for Continuing Medical Education) at **www.accme.org** and AAFP (American Association of Family Physicians) at **http://www.aafp.org/cme**

- Lawyers: CLE (Continuing Legal Education) at **www.cle.com**

- Respiratory Therapists: CoARC (Committee on Accreditation for Respiratory Care) at **www.coarc.com**

- Social Work: ABECSW (American Board of Examiners in Clinical Social Work) at **http://www.abecsw.org/**

12. *How does an organization become an accredited provider of professional continuing education hours?*

12. The organization must first meet the listed professional association's criteria to become an accredited provider. An application to become a provider of professional continuing education hours is completed and the appropriate fee included.

Professionals involved in the organization applying for provider status must hold the proper degrees in the profession involved.

13. *What requirements must be met for accredited approvers to approve professional continuing education hours?*

13. An organization seeking accreditation as an approver of professional continuing education in the profession identifies a separate, defined approver unit, which is administratively and operationally responsible for coordinating all aspects of the approval process.

Organizations seeking accreditation as approvers of continuing education must have the capacity and system in place to confer all categories of approval for which they are authorized.

14. *What exactly is needed by an approved provider to grant professional hours?*

14. The criteria for a teacher-directed program are that the educational activity involves participant attendance. Examples of these activities are conferences and workshops.

Providers design a learner-directed activity for completion, independently, at the learner's own pace and at a time of the learner's choice. The provider designs the educational activity and determines the amount of credit to be awarded. Examples of these activities include viewing videotapes or listening to audiotapes and completing posttest questions; accessing computer online activities; reading selected article(s) and completing posttest questions; and learning and practicing skills independently and seeking an instructor to evaluate a return demonstration.

The former learner-directed requirement for pilot testing has recently been replaced. "Contact hours are determined in a logical and defensible manner, consistent with the objectives, content, teaching-learning strategies, and target audience" (ANCC, **www.nursingworld.org/ancc/accred/approver/ appdxc.htm** on 11/05/01). This determination can be in the form of pilot testing but does not have to be.

15. What are the hallmarks of a well-designed online professional continuing education course?

15.

- Use learner-friendly Web page design, including consistent navigation icons and consistent placement from page to page, using easy-on-the-eye colors and visuals, directing the learner's eye consistently through the pages, keeping distractions at a minimum, and using appropriate fonts and font sizes.

- Keep scrolling and paging to a minimum.

- Keep important information at the top of course Web pages.

- Web pages content is easily viewed on both PC and Macintosh computers.

- Preview the course on all popular browsers to check for consistent function and appearance.

- Graphics are carefully used and file sizes kept to a minimum.

- Asynchronous student and teacher collaboration and discussion are included.

- Expert course facilitation is assured.

- Trust between all students and the teacher is ensured so that synchronous discussions are open and honest without fear of embarrassment or ridicule by others.

- Clear course schedules so learners know what they are to do at what time.

- Excellent materials that are easy to understand

- Good pedagogy

- Quality assurance through learner evaluation ensures any needed changes are made before the next course begins.

- Attention to disability issues when designing course Web pages and navigation

- Check all hyperlinks regularly to ensure that they remain active.

RESOURCES

American Association of Colleges of Nursing, Commission on Collegiate Nursing Education.
http://www.aacn.nche.edu/Accreditation/index.htm

American Nurses Credentialing Center. Selected glossary of accreditation terms.
http://www.nursingworld.org/ancc/accred/accrdorg/appd.htm

American Nurses Credentialing Center. Accreditation Eligibility Criteria.
http://www.nursingworld.org/ancc/accred/approver/2-2.htm

American Nurses Credentialing Center Commission on Accreditation. Appendix C: Criteria for approval as a provider of continuing education in nursing. *Manual for Accreditation as a Provider of Continuing Nursing Education 2001–2002*. Retrieved November 5, 2001, from
http://www.nursingworld.org/ancc/accred/approver/appdxc.htm

Division of Government of Public Affairs. (2000, March). *Developing a distance education policy for the 21ˢᵗ century.* Retrieved from **http://www.acenet.edu/washington/distance_ed/2000/03march/distance_ed.html**

Lynch, P., & Horton, S. Graphic design 101. *Web style guide.* Retrieved from
http://info.med.yale.edu/caim/manual/pages/graphic_design100.html

National Cancer Institute. Research-based Web design & usability guidelines.
http://usability.gov/guidelines/

National League for Nursing Accreditation Commission. **http://www.nln.ac.org**

Phillips, V. *The Virtual University Gazette's FAQ on distance learning on distance education, accreditation, and college degrees.* **http://www.geteducated.com/articles/dlfaq.htm#Q2**

Western Interstate Commission for Higher Education. *Principles of good practice for electronically offered academic degree and certificate programs.* **http://www.wiche.edu/telecom/projects/balancing/principles.htm**

Tinker, R. (2001, November). E-Learning quality: The Concord Model for learning from a distance. *Bulletin, 85*(628). Retrieved from **http://www.nassp.org/news/bltn_elearning1101.html**

Section 10:
Ethical/Legal Considerations

E-educators must be aware of the ethics and laws that are shaping the roles, rights, and responsibilities of e-educators and e-learners. This chapter serves as a primer for raising your consciousness about these issues. You will learn about your responsibilities for protecting copyright, how to manage intellectual property, what to be mindful of about the privacy of learners, and your responsibilities for protecting the rights of human subjects in e-learning research.

Chapter 34: Copyright and Intellectual Property Rights Issues

1. What is intellectual property?

1. Intellectual property allows people to own their creativity and innovation in the same way that they can own physical property. The owner of intellectual property can control and be rewarded for its use, and this encourages further innovation and creativity to the benefit of society.

2. What is the difference between copyright, trademark, design, and patent?

2. Copyright protects materials such as literary and artistic works, music, films, sound recordings, and broadcasts, including multimedia and software.

Trademark protects the brand identity of goods and services allowing distinctions to be made between different dealers of similar products.

Design protects shapes and appearances such as functional or aesthetically pleasing objects or surface decorations, patterns, or ornaments.

Patent protects inventions of new and improved products and industrial application processes.

3. What specifically is copyright?

3. Copyright gives specific economic rights to the creators of a wide range of material fixed in a tangible form. The Copyright Act of 1978 (as amended from 1976) grants specific rights to a copyright owner:

- the right to reproduce the copyrighted work

- the right to prepare derivative works based upon the work

- the right to distribute copies of the work to the public

- the right to perform the copyrighted work publicly

- the right to display the copyrighted work publicly

- the right to be identified as the creator or owner of the copyrighted work

- the right to object to the distortion or mutilation of the copyrighted work

4. What does copyright protect?

4. Copyright protects personal and group expression. Material protected by copyright is called a "work." Copyright protects works of literature, art, music, pantomimes, choreography, pictorial, graphic, and sculptural works, audiovisual works such as sound recordings, movies, videos, DVDs, broadcasts, and all online content.

Copyright does not protect ideas, names, titles, facts, short phrases, slogans, familiar symbols and designs, mere variations of typographic ornamentation, lettering, or coloring, listings of ingredients or contents, works consisting entirely of information that is common property and includes no original authorship, and blank forms.

5. *When exactly is a work copyright-protected?*

5. Copyright protection is automatically granted to every creative work the moment that work is fixed in a tangible form of any kind. For example, the answer to this question is considered copyrighted as soon as the words are typed into the word processing software program and saved.

6. *What works can be protected by copyright?*

6.
- Original literary works such as novels, newspaper articles, lyrics for songs, and instruction manuals

- Original software programs and HTML coding

- Original dramatic works, including dance and mime

- Original musical works

- Original artistic works such as paintings, drawings, engravings, sculptures, photographs, diagrams, maps, architecture, and works of artistic craftsmanship

- The typographical arrangements of published editions of literary, dramatic, or musical works

- Sound recordings in any form (e.g., audio cassette, compact discs, records) including recordings of other copyrighted works of music, literature, or other sounds

- Films, including videos and digital video discs (DVDs)

- Broadcasts and cable programs, including satellite and encrypted broadcasts

7. *How long does copyright protection last?*

7. Works originally created on or after January 1, 1978, are automatically protected from the moment of their creation in a fixed form. Works are ordinarily given copyright protection throughout the author's life plus an additional 70 years after the author's death. For works made for hire, and for anonymous and pseudonymous works (unless the author is revealed in U. S. Copyright

Office records), the copyright duration is 95 years from publication or 120 years from creation.

Works originally created before January 1, 1978, but not published or registered by that date are also automatically protected. The law provides that the copyright for works in this category cannot expire before December 31, 2002, and for works published on or before December 31, 2002, the term of copyright will not expire before December 31, 2047.

Works originally created and published or registered before January 1, 1978, had a copyright that lasted 28 years from the date the copyright was secured, and the copyright was renewable during the 28th year. The Copyright Act of 1976 extended the renewal term for these works from 28 to 47 years. In 1998, a revision to the law further extended the renewal term by an additional 20 years. Currently, the law provides for a copyright renewal term of 67 years and a total term of protection of 95 years for works in this category.

8. Does a work have to have a copyright mark visible to be copyright-protected?

8. Works created after January 1, 1978, do not need to be registered or even show the copyright notice in order to be protected under U. S. copyright law. The decision to include or omit the copyright notice is the responsibility of the copyright owner and does not require permission from or registration with the U.S. Copyright Office based in the Library of Congress in Washington, DC.

The copyright notice for visual works must contain:

1. The symbol © (the letter "C" in a circle) or the word "Copyright"

2. The year of first publication

3. The name of the owner of the copyright

For example © 2001 Linda Puetz or Copyright 2001 Linda Puetz

9. Are images, e-mail, discussion forums, HTML code, and Web pages on the Internet copyright-protected?

9. Yes, they are. Even if there is no copyright mark visible, all online images, Web pages, e-mail, discussion and chat room forums, Usenet messages, HTML code, ASCII files, sound files, graphics files, executable computer programs, news stories, novels, and screenplays are copyright protected because they are all recorded in a tangible way.

10. *If I work on an assignment during work hours, does the product belong to the organization or to me?*

10. If a copyrighted work is created as a "work for hire," the employer owns the copyright, unless a different written agreement has been made between the creator and employer. A work for hire is defined as material prepared by an employee within the scope of employment, or work specially ordered or commissioned for use as a contribution to a collective work, a translation, a compilation, an instructional text, a test, answer material for a test, a sound recording, or an atlas.

11. *Can I alter an original version or image enough for it to now belong to me?*

11. U.S. Copyright law is quite explicit that the making of what are called "derivative works"—works based or derived from another copyrighted work—is the exclusive province of the owner of the original work. This is true even though the making of these new works is a highly creative process. If you write a story using settings or characters from somebody else's work, you need that author's permission. The one major exception to this is parody. You are allowed to make fun of a copyrighted work because it is considered fair use. (See Question 13 for more on Fair Use.)

12. *How can I tell if something is copyright-protected?*

12. The copyright symbol © or Copyright with the year and owner's name may be present, but if the work was created or published after January 1, 1978, it does not have to have the copyright notice in order to be protected under the Copyright Act. If you can see it, touch it, or hear it, it is best to assume the work is copyrighted and ask for permission before using it.

13. *What is "fair use"?*

13. Fair use is a complex set of guidelines associated with copyright law. Fair use allows certain types of copying without permission so criticism, news reporting, teaching, or research will not be suppressed.

The Copyright Act of 1978 (as amended from 1976) defines four factors to be considered when deciding if a specific action is considered "fair use:"

- The purpose and character of the use, including whether such use is of commercial nature or is for nonprofit educational purposes

- The nature of the copyrighted work

- The amount and substantiality of the portion used in relation to the copyrighted work as a whole

- The effect of the use upon the potential market for or value of the copyrighted work

14. *If I completely cite the copyrighted material in my work, do I still need to obtain permission to use it?*

14. According to U. S. copyright law (US Code: Title 17, 2001), if you use material from a copyrighted work outside the exceptions for fair use, it is a violation of copyright even if you cite the material. To comply with the law, as it currently exists, permission must be obtained from the copyright owner to use the work, even if the work is appropriately credited.

15. *If I don't charge for it, is it all right to use a copyrighted work without permission?*

15. Copyright is violated whether you charge money or not. The kinds and amounts of legal damages awarded may be affected, but not the fact that copyright was violated. To make matters worse, you can be held responsible for significant monetary damages if the commercial value of the copyrighted work has been harmed after using it without the owner's permission (US Code: Title 17, Section 504. 2001).

16. *If I want to use a copyrighted document or image, how do I find out to whom it belongs?*

16. Look carefully and thoroughly throughout the work for authorship or publisher information. If there is no ownership information related to the work available, you can try contacting the person or organization that provided the work. You can also try searching for the work using an online resource like the Copyright Clearance Center or related Web sites to help find the true owner of the work.

17. *Where can I go to search for copyright information about specific documents, books, music, films, photographs, or digital images?*

17. For text: Copyright Clearance Center Online at: **http://www.copyright.com** is the best resource to find print and electronic rights to text.

For music: ASCAP (American Society of Composers, Authors, and Publishers) at: **http://www.ascap.com/**, BMI (Broadcast Music Incorporated) at: **http://bmi.com/home.asp**, and SESAC, Inc. at: **http://www.sesac.com** are the best sources to get permission to use music.

For Canadian copyrighted works: CANCOPY (Canadian Copyright Licensing Agency) at: **http://www.uniquename.com/cancopy/home.html** provides permission to use Canadian copyrighted works.

18. *How do I get permission to use copyrighted materials?*

18. Contact the copyright owner and request permission to use the work. Describe exactly what you are creating, the work's intended audience, and how you intend to use the owner's copyrighted work in your creation.

19. What can happen if I use someone's copyrighted work without permission and it is discovered?

19. It's up to the owner to decide what to do in that situation. Copyright law is mostly civil law. If you violate copyright you will usually get sued, not be charged with a crime. Statutory damage awards can range from $200 to $150,000 depending on the circumstances surrounding the violation (US Code: Title 17, Section 504, 2001). In the United States, commercial copyright violation involving more than 10 copies and valued over $2500 was recently made a felony.

20. Does my United States copyright protect my work outside the U.S.?

20. There is no such thing as an "international copyright" that will automatically protect a work throughout the entire world. Protection against unauthorized use in a particular country depends solely on the laws of that country. However, most countries do offer some protection to foreign works under certain conditions, and these conditions have been greatly simplified by international copyright treaties and conventions.

21. What are the specific intellectual property issues related to online learning?

21. One of the first steps an institution should take when developing a distance education policy is to review the institution's existing intellectual property policies and determine whether they need revision. An online learning policy will often involve patent, copyright, and software policies, and for some institutions, trademark, multimedia, and videotaping policies as well. Examination of these intellectual property policies often will encourage the institution to consider the relative balances between its various missions, including, for example, research, dissemination of knowledge, commercialization of technology, and public service. It is crucial to define in writing who owns the copyright for online education courses and related Web pages—the creator or the institution. Faculty issues may arise about how much teaching load credit will be given for teaching online and how online teaching may affect promotion and tenure.

Development of online learning brings another important issue into the open. Almost everything encountered online qualifies for copyright protection, including the text of Web pages, ASCII text documents, contents of e-mail, chat rooms, and Usenet messages, sound files, graphics files, executable computer programs, computer program listings, news stories, novels, and screenplays. Exceptions are online works that are known to be in the public domain. Public domain works include materials which were non-copyrightable to start with, works that lost their copyright protection, works that were created before January 1, 1978, that did not already have a valid copyright, all documents and publications of the U. S. federal government, works whose copyright expired, and works turned over to the public domain by their copyright owners. Care must be exercised in the creation of online education when using copyrighted materials already online, and in protecting the newly created copyrighted online education from illegal use by others.

RESOURCES

American Association of University Professors. AAUP Views on Distance Education and Intellectual Property. **http://www.aaup.org/govrel/distlern/deipdocs.htm**

BitLaw: A Resource on Technology Law. **http://www.bitlaw.com/copyright/index.html**

Copyright Web site. **http://www.benedict.com**

Developing a Distance Education Policy for 21st Century Learning. American Council on Education. Division of Government Public Affairs. March 2000. **http://www.acenet.edu/washington/distance_ed/2000/03march/distance_ed.html**

Intellectual Property. **http://www.intellectual-property.gov.uk**

Templeton, B. Ten Big Myths About Copyright Explained. **http://www.templetons.com/brad/copymyths.html**

U.S. Code: Title 17, Section 504 **at http://www4.law.cornell.edu/uscode/17/504.html**. Content last reviewed on 01/02/01.

U.S. Copyright Office, Copyright Basics. **http://www.loc.gov/copyright/circs/circ1.html#wccc**

Chapter 35: *Privacy*

1. What are the essential elements of online privacy?

1.
- The Web site has an online privacy policy.
- The privacy policy is easy to find, read, and understand.
- Every person must be given the choice to decide how private information about them may be used if the use intended is not related to the original purpose for the information.
- Organizations creating, maintaining, using, or disseminating individually identifiable information should take appropriate measures to ensure its reliability, take reasonable precautions to protect private information from loss, misuse or alteration, and take reasonable steps to ensure data collected are accurate, complete, timely, and used only for declared purposes.
- A process to address protection of data quality and steps to be taken if privacy is breached or data altered in any way.

2. What are the most effective ways to protect personal privacy online?

2.
- Look for privacy policies and read them.
- Get a separate e-mail account for personal e-mail.
- Remember that giving out information online means giving it to strangers.
- Clear the memory cache after browsing.
- Make sure online forms are secure.
- Reject unnecessary cookies.
- Use anonymous re-mailers.
- Encrypt your e-mail.
- Use anonymizers while browsing.
- Opt-out of third party information sharing.
- Use common sense, ask questions, and seek out resources.

3. If an online learner wishes to remain anonymous, what are the best ways to ensure anonymity will be protected?

3. The learner needs to:
- consistently use pseudonyms when online
- use anonymizer Web services
- install and use encryption software
- install and use re-mailer software
- reject unnecessary cookies

4. What is FERPA and how does it affect online privacy?

4. The Family Educational Rights and Privacy Act (FERPA) of 1974 maintains that any school, college, or university that receives federal funds has restrictions over the release of student records regardless of how the record is maintained or who maintains it. That includes electronic records that include confidential student information.

At institutions of higher education, only students can authorize the release of their educational records. This means that, in most cases, even a student's parent may not demand the release of the student's educational record. Teachers may not publicly post grades or test scores in a physical location or online without the student's permission.

There are some circumstances where educational records may be released without a student's permission. For instance, records may be disclosed to other school officials and teachers within the institution who are determined to have legitimate educational interests. An institution may also release educational records in response to a judicial order or a lawfully issued subpoena. Under limited circumstances, records may be released to appropriate parties in connection with an emergency—but only if the information is necessary to protect the health or safety of the student or other individuals.

5. What special privacy considerations should be employed for children?

5. Adults should:

- teach children NEVER to give out any personal information while online

- teach children to immediately leave a Web site that makes them uncomfortable or asks for information that is not supposed to be shared

- use software blockers that restrict or prohibit certain Web sites

- read each Web site's privacy policies related to children

- surf the Internet with children

- design Web pages that ask for private information to block those under 13 and/or require a parent's permission to log on

6. How can I protect my private materials from being read by others?

6. Using special software saving options and encrypting the materials are the most effective at protecting private materials from being read by others.

7. What is encryption?

7. Encryption is the conversion of data into a form that cannot be easily understood by unauthorized people.

8. Do my electronic communications belong to my employer or me?

8. If your electronic communications were created and sent through the employer's network or by using an employer-owned computer, then your electronic communications belong to your employer. Under these circumstances your employer has the right to open and read any communications you send.

If you own your computer and send electronic communications only from that system, you own those communications and no one else has the right to open and read them.

9. What are cookies?

9. A cookie is information within a very small file that a Web site puts on your computer's hard drive so that it can remember something about you if you return. Cookies are commonly used to rotate the banner ads that a site sends so that it doesn't keep sending the same ad as it sends you a succession of requested pages. Cookies can also be used to customize pages for you based on your browser type or other information you may have provided the Web site. Web users must agree to let cookies be saved for them, but, in general, cookies help Web sites to serve users better.

10. How can I explore the Internet without leaving private information behind?

10. You can use the ways to remain anonymous mentioned in Question 3. Also, your computer browser can be set to never accept Web site cookies or to prompt you when a Web site wants a cookie so you can say yes or no.

11. Does deleting my files from my hard drive or floppy disk guarantee they cannot be recovered?

11. Normally, deleting files from your hard drive or floppy disk means they can't be recovered. However, deleting items from your hard drive or floppy disk does not mean those files absolutely cannot be recovered. Given enough money and sufficient expert personnel, even completely erased hard drive files and floppy disk files can be recovered to a certain extent. To make recovery as difficult as possible, special software can be installed that lays nonsense data over parts of the hard drive or floppy disk. This makes it very hard to resurrect files no matter what recovery methods may be attempted.

12. How easy is it for someone to access my private information through the Internet?

12. In some cases, it is very easy for someone to access your private information on the Internet. It can be a frightening experience to put your own name in a browser and see what information can be found about you. Also there are many Web sites that specialize in finding persons when given the name, address, city, phone number, and/or e-mail address. For example, DocuSearch announces on its Web page, "DOCUSEARCH.COM is the place to find, locate & track down anybody! We offer locate searches, DMV driver & vehicle searches, telephone record searches, financial & bank searches, criminal & property records, plus hundreds of free searches" (Docusearch, 2001). It's very important to know the privacy and confidentiality policies of the Web pages you visit so that your private information isn't sold or given away without your knowledge.

13. What are some tools I can use to protect my online privacy?

13. Many software products exist to protect private information online. Privacy protection software products include encryption, advertisement blockers, anonymizers, browser testing, cookie management, file management, profile management, and spyware.

14. How does the Health Insurance Portability and Accountability Act (HIPAA) influence the privacy and confidentiality of healthcare information?

14. Without adequate privacy protections for private health information, individuals take steps to shield themselves from what they consider harmful and intrusive uses of their health information. Sometimes this omission can cause significant cost to their health. To address this problem, the government passed HIPAA in 1996 with implementation set for 2000. There have been implementation difficulties and the government has extended the implementation date several times.

HIPAA is designed to ensure each person has control over personal health information. Under HIPAA, individuals may request restrictions on treatment, payment, or healthcare related uses and disclosures of their private health information. However, a covered entity (e.g., hospital, physician's office) is not required to comply with these requests unless it explicitly agrees to do so. In all but the most unusual cases, it is likely that a covered entity will not choose to comply with individual requests for restrictions. Rather, it will direct patients to its Notice of Privacy Practices for an explanation of how their private health information will be used.

RESOURCES

CDT. Guide to On-line Privacy: **http://www.cdt.org/privacy/guide/basic/topten.html** and
http://www.cdt.org/resourcelibrary/Privacy/Tools/

DocuSearch. URL: **http://www.docusearch.com**

FTC. Keeping Kids Safe on the Internet. **http://www.kidsprivacy.com**

HIPAAdvisor: Legal Q&A. Can an Individual Against Unwanted PHI Uses?
http://www.hipaadvisory.com/action/advisor/HIPAAdvisor.htm

Maricopa Community College. A FERPA Primer. **http://www.dist.maricopa.edu/legal/ferparticle.html**

On-line Privacy Alliance. **http://www.privacyalliance.org/resources/ppguidelines.shtml**. 2001

TechTarget. Encryption definition. SearchSecurity.com.
http://searchsecurity.techtarget.com/sDefinition/0,,sid14_gci212062,00.html

TechTarget. Cookie definition. SearchSecurity.com.
http://searchsecurity.techtarget.com/sDefinition/0,,sid14_gci211838,00.html

Chapter 36: *Conducting Research and IRB Considerations*

1. What is the Helsinki Declaration?

1. The World Medical Association developed the Declaration of Helsinki as a statement of ethical principles to provide guidance to physicians and other participants in medical research involving human subjects. Medical research involving human subjects includes research on identifiable human material or identifiable data.

2. What is the Belmont Report?

2. The 1979 Belmont Report is the major ethical statement guiding human research in the United States. The Report established three ethical principles used as the framework for the protection of human subjects for both biomedical and behavioral research. Those principles are:

- respect for persons—respecting the autonomy of research subjects

- beneficence—the act of securing the well-being of research subjects

- justice—fairness in the distribution of the burdens and benefits of research

3. What are the important regulations and statutes that govern how human subjects research is conducted in the United States?

3. The primary federal regulations for the protection of human research subjects are housed within two government agencies. The Office of Human Research Protections is responsible for enforcing the Protection of Human Subjects Title 45 Code of Federal Regulations 46 and the Common Rule 45 CFR 46 Subpart A, and the Food and Drug Administration (FDA) enforces Protection of Human Subjects 21 CFR 50 and Institutional Review Boards 21 CFR 56.

4. What are the special considerations regarding human subjects in research?

4.
- Subject recruitment procedures

- Risk/benefit ratio

- Informed consent

- Subject vulnerability

- Investigator expertise

- Investigator conflicts of interest

- Research misconduct

5. What education is required by the U.S. Government in order to apply for National Institutes of Health (NIH) research grants?

6. What is an IRB?

7. What are the responsibilities of the Institutional Review Board in protecting the subjects of research?

5. In June 2000 the NIH Office of Extramural Research issued a requirement that all researchers conducting research involving human subjects with NIH funds must receive training on the protection of human subjects.

6. Persons conducting research involving human subjects have an ethical as well as professional, and in some cases legal, obligation to ensure the safety, protection, and rights of participants. The Institutional Review Board (IRB) is the official body within a research organization that defends the safety, protection, and rights of research participants.

7. The primary responsibility of the IRB is to review all research involving human subjects conducted at or sponsored by the institution regardless of the source of funding and ensure the research meets all federal and state guidelines. Areas commonly scrutinized by IRBs are:

- research and protocol design

- deciding if human subjects are involved

- informed consent to ensure the subject was not coerced

- special situations such as when research includes vulnerable subjects or research is done outside the United States

- deciding if the potential for benefit outweighs the potential for harm

- collecting and assessing research adverse events

- choosing whether the research protocol is exempt from IRB review

- review of previously approved protocols to ensure they are consistent with the original proposal

The IRB also establishes procedures for IRB initial and continuing review, approving research, reporting findings to the investigator and the institution, and determining which protocols need more than annual review.

8. What is informed consent/assent?

8. Except as provided by law, no investigator may involve a human being as a research subject unless the investigator has obtained the legally effective informed consent of the subject or the subject's legally authorized representative. Informed consent is not just a document that human subjects sign. Carefully establishing a well thought out process of informed consent goes much further to ensure that a true exchange of information occurs so the subject can voluntarily decide to participate or not participate in a research project.

Assent is consent to participate in research which is given by someone under 18 years of age. In this case, a parent or guardian must give informed consent as well.

9. What nine research education subject areas are highly recommended for all researchers, research administrators, and research staff by the U.S. Office of Research Integrity?

9.
- Data acquisition, management, sharing, and ownership
- Mentor/trainee responsibilities
- Publication practices and responsible authorship
- Peer review
- Collaborative science
- Human subjects
- Research involving animals
- Research misconduct
- Conflict of interest and commitment

10. How do I find existing online teaching resources for the responsible conduct of research?

10. The Office of Human Research Protections (OHRP) and the Office of Research Integrity (ORI) both have extensive lists of Web sites specializing in teaching the responsible conduct of research. Another way to find online teaching resources is to use a search engine. Good word combinations to use are "research education," "RCR education," "mandatory research education," and "required research education."

11. What are sanctions that may be imposed on an institution or individual for failure to provide sufficient protections to human subjects or animals participating in research?

11. For institutions with Health and Human Services grants, OHRP has a range of sanctions that may be imposed. If complaints are received from subjects, researchers, institutions, or publicized in media reports, OHRP assembles a compliance oversight evaluation team to investigate the institution's research division. Possible outcomes of the site visit are:

- a finding that no wrongdoing has been committed

- some of the protections offered by the institution may need to be strengthened

- the institution is not in compliance and corrective actions must be implemented

- the institution is not in compliance and affected research projects may continue

- the institution is not in compliance and some research projects will be halted

- the institution is not in compliance and all research projects will be halted

- an investigator or investigators are declared ineligible to participate in research

- the institution is declared ineligible to participate in research

12. *Learners in an online course take a survey as part of the course. Is IRB approval needed?*

12. If the survey results will not be published, and are a part of typical course and curriculum evaluation procedure then IRB approval is not necessary. However, if the survey results will be published, or reported to the public then IRB approval for the survey is necessary.

RESOURCES

Association for Assessment and Accreditation of Laboratory Animal Care. The Accreditation Program. **http://www.aaalac.org/accredit.htm**

Dunn, C., & Chadwick, G. (1999). *Protecting study volunteers in research.* Boston, MA: CenterWatch, Inc.

Institutional Animal Use and Committee. **http://www.iacuc.org/**

National Commission for the Protection of Human Subjects of Biomedical and Behavioral Research. *The Belmont report.* **http://ohrp.osophs.dhhs.gov/humansubjects/guidance/belmont.htm**

Office of Human Research Protections. Compliance Oversight Procedures. **http://ohrp.osophs.dhhs.gov/references/ohrpcomp.pdf**. URL:

Office of Research Integrity. RCR Education. **http://ori.dhhs.gov/html/programs/rcr_requirements.asp**

World Medical Association. Helsinki Declaration. **http://ohsr.od.nih.gov/helsinki.php3**

Index